THE POWER OF BODY AWARENESS

The Ultimate Guide to Relax and Loosen Your Body and Mind

Ready, Set, Wake Up Your Hidden Power!

Hideo Takaoka

THE POWER OF BODY AWARENESS

Published by Babel Press U.S.A.

This book was originally published in Japanese under the title
"身体意識を鍛える"
by Seishun shuppansha Ltd., Tokyo, Japan in 2003.

Author: Hideo Takaoka

Director: Tomoki Hotta

Translator: Rieko Sasaki
Coordinator: Junko Rodriguez
Formatting: Sota Torigoe

ISBN-10: 0983640238
ISBN-13: 978-0-9836402-3-3

Babel Corporation
Pacific Business News Bldg. #208,
1833 Kalakaua Avenue,
Honolulu, Hawaii 96815

Phone: (808) 946 - 3773
Fax: (808) 946 - 3993

Website: http://www.bookandright.com/

COPYRIGHT NOTICE

SAFETY NOTES

The exercises in this book are all mild workouts and designed with a strong attention to safety. However, depending on a practitioner's body condition, mental condition, way of practice, and environment of practice, it may create a risk of injury or accident. To avoid such a risk, choose safe and appropriate exercises, ways, and environment according to your own condition and circumstances. During your practice, be sure to release all the tension in your body. Practice softly and gently to avoid a risk of injury or accident.

If you experience any problems including suffering pain, dizziness, nausea, uncomfortable feeling, heaviness in the head, or lightheaded, etc., stop the practice immediately and ask for a doctor's consultation.

<IMPORTANT>

Health improvement effects of YURU EXERCISES (including the exercises in this book) have been verified by universities and research organizations in Japan under their study and research. However, if you have an issue with your health, you should get your doctor's approval before beginning and practice under the doctor's guidance.

DISCLAIMER

Table of Contents

THE POWER OF BODY AWARENESS

Introduction

Michael Jordan, Muhammad Ali, Jack Nicklaus, Ingemar Stenmark, Usain Bolt, Ichiro. You might have heard these names. They are all super stars in the sports world of the 20th and 21st centuries. If I tell you "It is possible that you can have the subconsciousness that supports the same excellent quality of body and mind capability like them," how would you feel? "You must be kidding!" "I just have an ordinary life. I don't need that kind of ability." Perhaps many people would say so.

Yes, unless you are trying to be a professional athlete, our daily lives do not usually require the special capabilities shown by Michael Jordan, Usain Bolt, or Ichiro. Such abilities are particularly needed for success in their fields. We have almost no need or opportunity to use the movements or muscular power—their particular body and mind capabilities—as is.

However, think about their relaxed arm movements, smooth footwork, and strong stable body axes. In other words, look at how effectively they use their bodies. They are 'body usage experts.' How would you feel if you had the same 'body usage' ability; if you could perform wonderful efficient movements just like them in your own circumstances, in your own life activities? Walking, going up and down stairs, driving a car, using a computer, carrying things, cooking, cleaning, and more and more. Don't you think even such daily activities can be done more easily, efficiently, comfortably, and beautifully?

When I looked at the core elements of the body usage experts from this point of view, I realized surprisingly that there are 'seven secrets of body usage' that applied to all of them. Here, I call them the 'seven gokui.' Gokui is a Japanese word that is often translated as 'secrets,' 'hints,' 'magic,' keys,' 'tips,' etc. However, in my body awareness concept, the term 'gokui' refers to 'ultimate awareness.' It represents the state of body awareness in which the structures and functions of the body and mind are operating at maximal effectiveness.

This is not just a story about athletes. The seven gokui applies to the top performing people in many fields. They apply even in various aspects of Japanese traditional culture including martial arts, Zen, classical dance-drama performing arts such as Kabuki, Noh chant, and other traditional dance, or shamisen (a three-stringed musical instrument). If we look across at other professionals such as musicians, artists, chefs, hairdressers, as well as scientists, doctors, teachers, business executives and others, the seven gokui can be seen in top performing people in any and all fields.

So, what are the seven gokui? What is currently lacking in your body? What is the obstacle to mastering the gokui of the experts' body usage?

This book reveals these seven gokui and provides training methods to master them. After I studied a variety of physical training methods from all ages and cultures as well as the physical abilities of animals (especially fish) for decades, these methods were born as "YURU EXERCISES." The YURU EXERCISES were created based on the theory and techniques of Japanese traditional martial arts. Together with the essence from those, multiple techniques are integrated including exercises to loosen and relax your body with body rubbing and shaking and those to change your body and mind dramatically using gentle humor and Japanese onomatopoeia.

You may feel depressed when you read the word 'exercise.' But the YURU EXERCISES I introduce to you here are very easy and very little effort is needed. Just incorporate them into your daily life. You will notice many benefits and find a superior cost-performance.

The benefits will not only be from the physical aspect. You can expect many kinds of mental benefits as well with each body awareness type. Also, having a comfortable and efficient body will positively affect your mental state. You will no longer worry about the small stuff, but rather be more stable and see things in a wider and higher point of view. You will be more motivated and energized to move forward to your goals.

In this book, twelve basic YURU EXERCISES for developing all body awareness types and another twelve YURU EXERCISES for strengthening each of the seven body awareness types are introduced. Try the basic YURU EXERCISES first. Floor YURU and Sitting YURU are especially easy for everyone regardless of age and gender, and tremendous benefits can be expected to enhance your health. YURU EXERCISES are designed to create the 'relaxed and loosened body and mind' that you must obtain to develop the body awareness, and also simultaneously to develop and strengthen the body awareness itself.

Therefore, even if you think "I am not so interested in the body awareness," if you keep working on the Basic YURU EXERCISES, you will find you can easily recover from fatigue, cope well with stress, and have less risk of injuries or disease.

If you are interested in the body awareness itself, try the individually designed YURU EXERCISES for each body awareness type. With the appropriate approach and practice, you can expect various benefits depending on the body awareness types, such as you can begin to see things from a wider and higher point of view, have a greater presence of mind, or be more passionate, active, and positive.

We are currently working on the official website of YURU EXERCISES (http://yuruexercise.net/). It will provide you with many useful topics and information including features and benefits of YURU EXERCISES and medical scientific measurement data from the studies we have conducted. For those who wish to practice YURU EXERCISES in full scale or those who wish to teach YURU EXERCISES, this site will be helpful to watch practical training videos and see guidelines of teaching and studying instructions of YURU EXERCISES. (This site is planned to open after October 2014.)

I hope you will master the seven gokui (ultimate body awareness) and the YURU EXERCISES to enjoy a more comfortable life, both mentally and physically.

Hideo Takaoka

Chapter 1

Where do efficient bodies and economical movements come from?

The common points held by top performing people; Ichiro, Tiger Woods, Michael Jordan, etc.

In the 21st century, what the body requires is changing!

People's attention to the human body is getting much more acute nowadays. More people are interested in their physical abilities and functions. As if in response to this, a new concept of the body has arisen in the 21st century. In brief, the 20th century concept was an approach from the aspect of energy. What we discussed as the main focus was muscular power, whole body endurance, and maximal oxygen intake. How much power can a body produce instantaneously? How long can it maintain that power? We had focused on these points to find the main reason why people had differences in the abilities and functions of their bodies. Here, I am not just talking about professional athletes. Even at ordinary gyms, muscle training was very popular using barbells, aerobic-bikes, or other various machines. These help increase muscular output power or the whole body endurance. The 20th century was the heyday of this kind of training.

Towards the end of the century, this concept was being questioned in the advanced sport science field. People started thinking that the energy system such as muscle mass or the whole body endurance cannot maximize the abilities, functions, or operations of human bodies just by improving physical skills, which are abilities to use such an energy system.

Here are some well-known athletes: Michael Jordan (US NBA basketball player), Ingemar Stenmark (Swedish skier), Bonnie Blair (US speed skater who took five Olympic gold medals), Michael Phelps (US swimmer), Ichiro (Japanese baseball player who blasted the single-season hit record in the US Major League), Tiger Woods (US golfer), Usain Bolt (Jamaicans sprinter), and more and more can be listed.

During the intensive studies of these people's body usage and performances, their physical abilities could not be fully explained from the aspect of energy only. We are beginning to realize that there is something special that is controlling the abilities of the human body.

So, what is that something, which is not energy or physical skills?

I believe that it is the body awareness. It is beyond physical skills − the undifferentiated body-mind ability − that exists deep in our bodies and minds. Times have changed from the 20th century, the age of energy and physical skills to the 21st century, the age of the body awareness − the profound body-mind ability.

You can hang up your laundry on Ichiro's thrown ball

Let's talk about what the undifferentiated body-mind ability is. Here is the very best person who can describe this. Ichiro, the US major league baseball player. Especially looking at the time of his heyday, breaking George Sisler's single-season hit record, he is best example to explain this undifferentiated body-mind ability. Let's take a close look at him.

First, remember how well he played in US Major League games. Many people used to say his batted ball is 'the fastest in the entire league.' We can surely say his incredibly accurate and speedy throwing from outfield was top of the League. Lou Piniella, the former manager of Seattle Mariners, the club to which Ichiro belonged, used to say in praise, "You can hang up your laundry on Ichiro's thrown ball." This humorous quip suggests that Ichiro's ball line looked just like a very tightly stretched clothesline.

But actually there is a deeper meaning here. What kind of line do you imagine of the drawn clothesline? I guess you would think something very straight sideways or something with the center part hanging down a little. If you throw a ball far, it follows a gentle arch. But what Piniella said meant Ichiro's ball followed an upside down arch. You may understand how sharp and fast it is and even that it was a ball with a backspin.

Ichiro's throwing, which has been described as a 'laser beam', is truly super, but his batted ball also tends to follow a very sharp and straight line. US sports journalists and Major League commentators were saying in chorus that his batted ball speed was maybe number one in the Major League. Because it is difficult to accurately measure the actual speed of batted balls, it would be impossible to perfectly compare Ichiro with others. Even so, the fact is many baseball experts have recognized his super-fast batted balls. This means there is no doubt that he ranks among the best in the league.

Now Ichiro is in his 40s. Although his performance is not as impressive as that in his prime, he is still very active with almost no major injuries or physical problems at his age. Ichiro can be considered as one of the great athletes who can define a highly developed body awareness.

What is the key point so far? Take account of all of the above, then think about Ichiro's body once again.

For example, compare Ichiro's body size with that of his other teammates when they are all standing around in the dugout. The size difference is just like a kid with adults. Ichiro looks like a thin 10 or 11-year-old boy.

If the other players' body fat percentages were 30% or so, the story would be totally different. But they are all Major League players who have been well trained. For most of them, the body fat percentage is probably 10% or less. Their muscle mass (amount of muscle) is enormous. In proportion to this, their muscle force should be very high. From the viewpoint of energy, Ichiro's level is way below them. Plus, they are, of course, not amateur players. They have played a lot since they were small kids and their skills are at the highest level. Including the Minor League, the total number of the players will be far more compared to the Japanese professional baseball league. The major league teams' members are all the best of the baseball elite. Among those people, Ichiro who has less muscle has shown us top-level performances in all categories including offense, defense, and base running. That is incredible.

How did Ichiro achieve such high performance?

Think of it this way: If using the 20th century concept, the speed of a batted ball would be proportional to the speed of the bat swing. Thus, it is important how fast your arms and torso move. → You must move your mass fast. → You must have stronger muscles to increase the total muscle mass.

If this were an absolute requirement, the batted balls of Ichiro, a player with less muscle mass, would not be faster than those of other players with more muscle mass. Then, how can Ichiro beat the others?

The secret is based on three main points:

The first point is balance. In order to keep balance, a center axis is required similar to the axis of a wheel or the axis of a spinning top. Ichiro's core axis must be very accurate and stable to keep his body in balance. Also none of the energy generated by this well-balanced body is wasted.

The second point is to use the potential of many muscles all over the body. A human body consists of about 200 bones and 500 muscles. In the case of Ichiro, his speed is compiled by using many of those bones and muscles to great effect. In contrast, there are players who are massively built but their batted balls are not as fast. The addition of power and speed has not made enough of a difference in their bodies. They use limited muscles such as the ones in their hands or arms but cannot fully use other muscles such as those located in their torso. Compared to Ichiro, this kind of player cannot use the energy that could have been generated by the under-used parts of their body.

The third point is that nothing works as a brake in his body. Do you know a muscle has a role as an accelerator to produce speed, and simultaneously also provides resistance? Many players other than Ichiro have accelerator muscles but brake (resistance) muscles as well. Therefore they use both kinds of muscles at the same time when batting, running, and throwing. But Ichiro can completely control and avoid using the muscles that would work as a brake.

In the 20th century sports world, people simply thought that if a player had strong massive muscles as well as basic techniques, his throw and batted ball would be faster. Thus, when sports scientists were asked by athletes for training to improve their abilities, the scientists used to create a training regime that focused on strengthening particular muscles to be beneficial for the respective sport. Furthermore, they would focus on spending a lot of time for running or riding an aerobic-bike to increase whole body endurance.

However, if you look at Ichiro, it is obvious that such a kind of training cannot improve the real body functions. No more of the 20th century's age of energy and physical skills. In the 21st century, we are now at the age of body awareness—the profound ability of body and mind.

You can use your body more efficiently!

So now we have to think about how we can develop body abilities like the ones

Ichiro has. That's because, as you have seen, it is cost-efficient if high performance can be obtained from a small resource such as Ichiro's body.

Put body size on the bottom of a fraction and put performance (results) on top. This is called the performance weight ratio. In the case of Ichiro, it can be an amazing number. Assuming his batted ball is 111 mph, this speed should be equal to 125 mph or more for larger and heavier body batters. As just described, a body with the highly developed body awareness can be described as a 'highly efficient body.'

Then, what are the benefits when you have a highly efficient body? Even with a low body resource, high performance can be achieved. This is easy to understand. But the first thing you would feel when you have a highly efficient body is how comfortable it is.

Imagine there are two bicycles, A and B, in front of you. A is nicely maintained. You can ride it smoothly and comfortably from the very first pedal stroke. In contrast, B is rusty and in poor condition. It is really heavy and the power generator for its light is rubbing on the wheel and can't be released. Even worse, it makes a squeaky noise at each pedal stroke.

Think about riding these two bicycles to the train station a mile or two away. A person who rides on A must be very comfortable because the bike feels so smooth to ride. As you might have experienced, your stress will be gone with this nice bicycle. Riding on a slight downhill would make you exclaim, "Yee-ha!"

How about B? It takes so much energy for just one pedal stroke. It is very heavy and makes unpleasant noise. Your stress level just goes up. And other cyclists riding on well-maintained bicycles keep passing you on the left and right. You would feel embarrassed and want to find somewhere to hide.

In our bodies, a similar thing is happening. An efficient body, which means a high quality body with excellent body awareness, gives you the same sensation as you get from the nicely maintained bicycle A. Whereas a low quality body with lack of body awareness, even if it's a well-trained muscular body, is the same thing as bicycle B. Just walking increases your stress at each step. You cannot hear the squeaky noise from your body, but your body parts are actually scraping each other.

Which is your body?

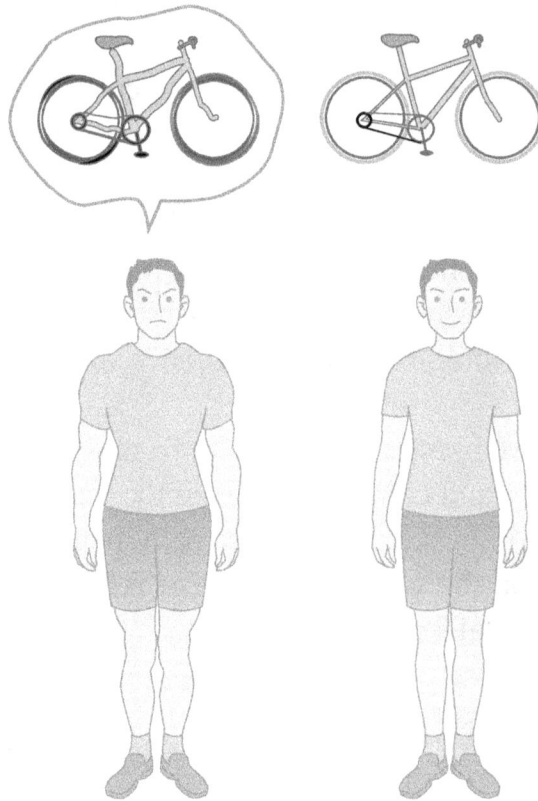

The difference between a bicycle and the human body is you cannot easily re-place your body. If it's a bicycle, the owner of bicycle B can borrow bicycle A from his friend. You can experience both the comfort and discomfort of the two types of bicycles. However, you have made the current state of your body over a long period of time. The daily change is very small. Because it cannot be compared and veri-fied like the bicycles, it would be hard to feel the difference even when your body is rusty and in poor condition.

Most of our bodies are probably the same as bicycle B compared to Ichiro. This may sound shocking to you, but the fact is almost 100% of people who are not do-ing any sports, martial arts, dance, or exercises such as Yoga or Qigong, etc., have type B bodies. Even for people who do sports or exercise regularly, more than 99% of those people are also type B. This is the case, because compared to Ichiro, even most Major League players are also type B.

Nobody wants to ride on the bicycle B. You must want to have a comfortable type A body rather than an unpleasant type B. But as you know, a human body cannot be replaced. So you have to fix and improve your body on your own. Are you sure? Is it possible to change my body to the one like Ichiro? You might ask these questions. The answer is YES.

I have talked about bicycles as an example, but the structure and mechanism of the human body is way more complicated than a bicycle. Getting comfortable is not as easy as performing maintenance on your bicycle. Then, what are the methods to maintain a complicated human body?

Magical awareness in your body

Have you ever heard of 'seichu-sen'? Seichu-sen is a Japanese word that means the vertical straight centerline that goes right through the middle of the human body from the top of the head to the bottom of the feet. This word is often used in the field of martial arts. Some of you readers might have heard of it because martial arts are very popular worldwide these days.

The next question is; how about the word 'tanden'? Tanden is also a Japanese word. In Oriental medicine, the tanden is considered to be the energy center of the whole body located below the navel. It is used for not only martial arts but also for Japanese traditional performing arts, Zen, Qigong, or Chinese martial arts. Thus, more people may know tanden than seichu-sen.

Now, how about these expressions? "He has a stable mind at his core," "He has guts," "He is gutsy." There may not be many people who have heard of seichu-sen or tanden. But there must be many people who know and use the words 'core' or 'guts.'

Seichu-sen and tanden are thought to improve human body abilities to the maximum and develop its wonderful functions. In Japan, through hundreds of years, many people have realized, approved, and verified the effectiveness and existence of seichu-sen and tanden. However, I have never ever heard any explanations of what they actually are.

About 40 years ago, when I was 20, I was very interested in seichu-sen and tanden and studied them in earnest. But all I could find was that seichu-sen or tanden is something magical or mystical. For example, tanden is located in the lower abdomen. It is said that you can feel a sense of stability and fulfillment there. A person who has tanden is aware of it in his body. People around such a person often say "That person has tanden." However, anatomically, there is nothing there other than the bowels. It is unsubstantial, but it surely exists. So what is it? This was my first question.

And I had another question. Is seichu-sen or tanden used only by Japanese people? Again, seichu-sen is a line going straight up and down through your body. This word is used in the world of Japanese martial arts and traditional performing arts. I was wondering if there was anything like this for other sports or in western cultures?

I brought this question to a martial arts teacher. He said "seichu-sen is typically used for martial arts only." I also asked a teacher of Japanese sword-fighting. He gave me the same answer. Then I asked a baseball coach. "When a human is standing, is there anything like a line going straight up and down through the body?" Can you guess what he answered? He said "That must be the body axis. We use it for baseball." Also, the answer from a golf instructor was like this, "That is the axis. In the field of golf, everybody says so." Both baseball and golf are sports that came from the western culture. But something similar to seichu-sen apparently exists in those fields, too.

Furthermore, I also asked a sister of my friend who was a classical ballet instructor. She said "Yes, we have that line in our field. We call it the center." I was amazed and asked again to make sure. "That center is the same as an axis or body axis in other sports, right?" She replied "Although 'center' may be used for modern ballet as well, this word must be originally and typically used for classical ballet."

I went back to the people in martial arts and told them about this. But they could not accept the idea that the center for ballet is the same as the seichu-sen for martial art. However, I was sure that seichu-sen in martial arts, body axis in baseball, axis in golf, and center in ballet were all the same thing. It is because when I asked the location of the line, everyone first pointed to the tip of head and explained that the line goes straight through the center of body from here.

The structure of the human body is the same for everyone. The location of the line is the same, too. Its shape is also the same. Therefore, that line must be the same thing but people just call it differently according to their field. That was my conclusion.

Discovery of body awareness

So, what are these things? Anatomically, no seichu-sen or tanden can be found as a specific type of organ shaped like a line or ball. But they are considered as something very important in various fields including martial arts, performing arts, and sports. If you have one, your body usage can be very flexible and reasonable. You can also feel the sense of stability and fulfillment mentally. These things are surely true.

What is this thing that is intangible but exists as if it is there, controlling the movements and the mind of a human?

It is human's 'awareness.' The thoughts you have in your mind are your awareness. But the awareness of 'seichu-sen' or 'tanden' is different. It is an awareness which surely exists in your body. So, I have called it 'body awareness.' In short, 'axis,' 'body axis,' 'seichu-sen,' and 'tanden' are all a type of 'body awareness.'

Now let's think back to the example of the bicycles. A human body cannot be separated like the parts of the bicycle. For example, unlike the saddle on the bicycle, hip joints are not connected to the body with a removable bolt. Even if hip joints are not symmetry aligned, or the spine is curved with scoliosis, it cannot be fixed as easily as fixing a frame or an axle of the bicycle's wheel. That is why the human body has a profound mechanism to keep balance of every part. This mechanism is body awareness.

A human body requires guidelines

Here is an example. If body awareness of 'a line that goes straight up and down through the body' is created in the same way as seichu-sen, what will happen to you?

First, that line will work as a guideline. You can stand up straighter. Imagine you are a marionette manipulated by a string. If you have an image that someone is pulling the strings from above, you can stand straighter and more beautifully as if your body is smoothly growing upward. This guideline allows you to spend less effort to keep balance. Your body will be correctly aligned without any problems such as your left shoulder is lower than the right shoulder, or your hip joints are leaning. As a matter of course, not just when standing but also when walking, by following this guideline you can keep your balance without using any extra energy.

However, in order to walk straight, a vertical guideline is not enough. Walking means going forward. If you have a horizontal guide line as well, you can walk unswervingly. In fact, there is a body awareness of the horizontal straight line, too.

I call this line 'the laser.' For body awareness of the vertical line mentioned above, I call it 'the center.'

Guidelines for walking

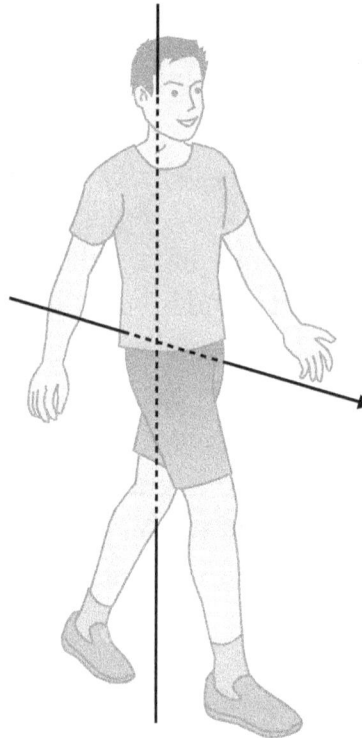

The body awareness of the vertical and horizontal lines can be guidelines. It will change your walking from ordinary movements to excellent movements. If these guidelines work at various times in your daily life or when you do sports, it will be obvious that your body quality will improve significantly compared to the situation where you have no guidelines at all. Body awareness works like this. It will improve your body operations, performances, and the quality of your body itself.

Now let's compare the bicycle and your body again. In the case of the bicycle, you can adjust the angle of each part, such as the handlebars, freely and appropriately and fix it firmly with bolts or nuts. You can ride on that bicycle smoothly and straight.

However, in the case of the body, you have no maintenance person. Even if such a person existed, each part of your body would start losing its balance immediately after the adjustment. The body cannot be fixed using bolts or nuts. The human body is not a machine. It is a living system. There is always the possibility that the positional relationship of each part of the body will go wrong second by second and foot by foot.

Therefore, we need something that can always fix the deviation and can align all parts of the body appropriately. That is one of the important natures of body awareness. People who are like Ichiro have highly developed body awareness. That is why they can use their bodies very efficiently just like riding on the well maintained bicycle.

Three requirements to produce Ichiro's power

1) Balance

First of all, let me talk about Ichiro's good balance. As mentioned above, it is important to have a core line at the center of the body. Ichiro can stand and move with great balance because his body awareness, 'center', the core line going straight up and down through his body, is well developed and because he uses the center as a guideline.

The human body is an indeterminate form consisting of many parts. Roughly, there are 200 bones that are organically connected to each other by about 500 muscles. Each joint connects bone-to-bone. Joints and bones are moving all the time. A human body does not remain fixed like a building. The center is the guideline to stand straight and accurately; for correlating bone-to-bone and bone-to-muscle in the correct way.

Think about building a tower. First, you place the support pillar in the center. Next, while using the pillar as a guideline, the surroundings will be built. Sometimes, the pillar is removed after the surroundings are done. In that case, the pillar was surely a guideline.

One of the famous Japanese architectural designs, the five-story pagoda, has endured the hard weather of wind, rain and snow for hundreds of years. It is well known as a strong architecture against earthquakes and typhoons. Some of the five-story pagodas do not have a thick support pillar. When this kind of pagoda was built, a long bamboo pole or a string with a balance weight was used as a guideline instead of the center pillar. This is the same system of guidelines that we use to keep our balance. Having an evenly aligned balance about the center means your muscles have no unnecessary tension. This further makes your body nice and loose. You can make various movements efficiently.

2) Dispersion and addition

The second secret that Ichiro has is that he can use the many parts of the muscles and bones in his body. This is actually because the center is working.

Muscles are activated in the area where your body awareness is developed. For example, let's think about our hands. You must have stronger awareness in your hands than feet. Do you know why? That certain parts of body can work better than other parts means the body awareness of the more efficient part is developed that much more. If you are right-handed, the body awareness of your right hand is more developed than that in your left hand. If you compare your chest and back, the body awareness of your chest should be stronger.

This means that body awareness always exists in the area where you can use your body parts well. The activated muscle controlled by body awareness will be fully relaxed when necessary. When it is necessary to produce power, it will immediately contract.

The center is the strong body awareness of the line going straight from the very top of the head to the bottom of the feet which coordinates the whole body. It is located in the area close to your spine. In other words, if you have awareness there, your inner muscles connected to each of the 26 vertebrae will be activated. As a result, all these muscles will quickly loosen in an appropriate order when relaxation is needed. In contrast, they will quickly contract in an appropriate order when power needs to be produced.

If each one of the bones and each one of the small muscle groups are nicely separated and move smoothly and flexibly with each other, the muscles located in between each of the body parts will have enough space for contraction and expansion. They can quickly contract as necessary. This makes it possible for you to pull out the hidden potentials that many muscles have and enables you to use your body where all the produced energies are maximally added. In academic parlance, I call this body usage 'dispersion and addition.'

Even with a small muscle mass, this body usage can create overwhelmingly higher performance than the athletes whose trunk is stiff like a box. When you look at Ichiro, his body is nice and loose. In all the situations of defense, offense, and base running, all the parts of his body, from head to feet, are separated but working harmoniously. He can use them separately, on and off, efficiently, quickly and strongly.

3)   Control of resistance (or 'brake') muscles

Why can Ichiro create the status of 'no resistance in the body'? The reason is Ichiro has a highly developed body awareness that activates his hamstrings and gluteus maximus muscle. I call this body awareness 'uratenshi' (back push). I will explain more about this awareness in the next chapter. But because of this body awareness, you can use your hamstrings efficiently as an accelerator but avoid using the quadriceps, which can be a resistance muscle (brake muscle).

When Ichiro runs to first base after his batting as well as when he dashes to steal a base, he mainly uses his hamstrings in which the uratenshi is working well. When you see Ichiro's batting, it looks like he starts running while batting. But Ichiro says, "I have never ever done it like that." He completes his batting and then he starts running. Even so, the audience sees that he starts running while batting. He can make such smooth seamless movements.

By thinking about that point, let's compare Ichiro with other players. If you focus on the thigh muscles, many players try to start to run at the state where their front thigh muscles (quadriceps) are working. But the quadriceps is a muscle that resists and disrupts the attempt to move forward. Therefore, you have to overcome that resistance first. Otherwise, you cannot move fast.

In the case of Ichiro, his quadriceps are released and relaxed from the beginning. He uses his hamstrings from the beginning. That is why he can dash forward with no resistance applied. As described, Ichiro has highly developed body awareness in his core centerline and hamstrings. Because this awareness is more accurate, much sharper and stronger than others, he can perform his super body movements.

Reflecting back on myself, when I was an undergraduate 40 years ago, I noticed 'seichu-sen and tanden are all awareness that exists with a physical body.' After that, I took a major of sports science in a master's degree course and studied intensively about human bodies, movements, and abilities. I have also studied the body awareness such as 'seichu-sen' or 'tanden' thoroughly. As a result, I have found that there are many more types of body awareness functions and shapes in our body system even though they do not have particular names like 'seichu-sen.'

In the next chapter, I introduce the 'seven gokui (seven body awareness types)' to you. These are the keys to allow you to have efficient body usage.

Chapter 2

The Seven Gokui of Experts' Body Usage Revealed

Body Awareness revives your body and mind

Seven Body Awareness Types

Body Awareness		
1	**Center**	

Body Sense	Benefits
•Stand straight •Higher eye level •Large inhalations •Don't worry about small things •Sharp sensations •Cool looking •Stable core	•The centerline of gravity can be used •The psoas major muscle always works •Activates hamstrings •Better balance of each body part •Creates the axis for the rotational movement

Deficiency Symptoms	Who has developed awareness?
•Overstrain, try too hard •Lower center of gravity •Narrower vision •Worry about small things	•Ichiro (Baseball) •Tiger Woods (Golf) •Michael Jordan (Basketball) •Kikunosuke Onoe (Kabuki) •Sylvie Guillem (Ballet) •Kim Yu-Na (Figure skating) •Carl Lewis (Track and field) •Ingemar Stenmark (Skiing) •Ted Williams (Baseball) •Anton Geesink (Judo) •Yasuhiro Yamashita (Judo)

Body Awareness		
2	**Lower Tanden**	

Body Sense	Benefits
•Steady mind •Deeper inhalations •Robust sensation	•Activates iliopsoas muscle and diaphragm •Promotes abdominal respiration •Loosens shoulder muscles •Controls automatic nerves
Deficiency Symptoms	**Who has developed awareness?**
•Easy to become upset •Restless mind •Short temper •Easy to get stressed out •Easy to be short of breath	•Jack Nicklaus (Golf) •Muhammad Ali (Boxing) •Yasuhiro Yamashita (Judo)

Body Awareness		
3	**Middle Tanden**	

Body Sense	Benefits
•Passionate •Thrilled •Motivated •Active •Excited •Positive	•Activates heart and arteries •Raises heart rate •Stimulates sympathetic nerves
Deficiency Symptoms	**Who has developed awareness?**
•No motivation •Cannot love people •No passion •Gloomy •Depressed	•Steve Jobs (Entrepreneur and inventor) •Lady Gaga (Singer and songwriter) •Bruce Lee (Actor) •Tony La Russa (Baseball manager) •John F. Kennedy (Politician) •Babe Ruth (Baseball) •Alberto Tomba (Skiing) •Muhammad Ali (Boxing)

Body Awareness	
4 **Arch**	

Body Sense	Benefits
•Love •Cooperative •Friendly •Trusting •Clear feeling (no worries or concerns)	•Become passionate •Be gentle to others •Be treated gently by others •Become popular •Higher communication ability

Deficiency Symptoms	Who has developed awareness?
•Sad •Poor social skills •Unfriendly •Isolated •No confidence	•Lady Gaga (Singer and songwriter) •Steve Jobs (Entrepreneur and inventor) •Michael Jordan (Basketball) •Lionel Messi (Soccer) •Joe DiMaggio (Baseball) •Babe Ruth (Baseball)

Body Awareness	
5 **Vest**	

Body Sense	Benefits
•Relaxed upper body (shoulders and arms) •No stiff shoulders •Lower brain fatigue •Easier fine hand movements	•Higher flexibility on the base of arms •Reduces burden on the brain •Activates shoulder blades

Deficiency Symptoms	Who has developed awareness?
•The whole upper body gets stiff including the parts of shoulders, back underarms, chest •Difficulty breathing •Feel fatigue in arms, hands, and brain	•Greg Maddux (Baseball) •Rickson Gracie (Mixed martial arts) •Michael Phelps (Swimming) •Björn Borg (Tennis) •Masutatsu Oyama (Karate) •Clayton Kershaw (Baseball) •Joe Frazier (Boxing)

Body Awareness		
6	**Uratenshi (Back Push)**	

Body Sense	Benefits
•High center of gravity •Feel supported from the back •Quick and easy walking •Feel positive •Light footwork	•Activates upper hamstrings •Quick start •Strong forward power •Relaxes quadriceps

Deficiency Symptoms	Who has developed awareness?
•Too lazy to walk •Inactive •Difficult to start •Cannot face forward	•Mao Asada (Figure skating) •Cristiano Ronaldo (Soccer) •Naoko Takahashi (Marathon) •Yasuhiro Yamashita (Judo) •Usain Bolt (Track and field) •Paula Radcliffe (Marathon) •Rickey Henderson (Baseball) •Bonnie Blair (Speed skating)

Body Awareness		
7	**Laser**	

Body Sense	Benefits
•Act accurately and stay focused on target •Sharp insights •Go straight •Stable axis	•Creates straight anterior direction line •Improves balance for forward motion •Creates clear and stable direction

Deficiency Symptoms	Who has developed awareness?
•Incoherent •Lose direction •Unstable movements or actions	•Ichiro (Baseball) •Tiger Woods (Golf) •Usain Bolt (Track and field) •Michael Phelps (Swimming) •Cristiano Ronaldo (Soccer) •Tyson Gay (Track and field) •Maurice Greene (Track and field) •Nolan Ryan (Baseball) •Roger Clemens (Baseball)

Type 1: Center

The first body awareness I am going to discuss is 'the center' that I talked about in the example of Ichiro. Think of the center as an academic inclusive term applied to 'seichu-sen,' 'axis,' or 'body axis.' The center is a line that goes straight up and down through the body.

Look at the illustrations below. The center goes through several points in the body; slightly behind the middle of the head (hyakue -acupuncture point), slightly in front of the anus (perineum), in between the ankles when your legs are evenly aligned and straight, and slightly in front of the spine as a point inside the torso.

The location of the center

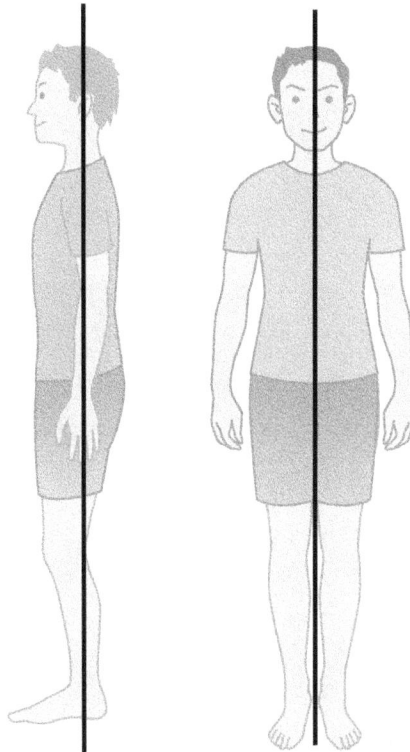

To be exact, the spine draws an S curve. So the center goes through the middle of the spine where it curves forward, and touches slightly in front of the spine where it curves backward. The center is not exactly the same as the line of the spine.

The center stretches deep down towards the middle of the earth. I call that point the 'chi-shin (earth core).' Also, the center stretches up to the sky. Because it is awareness, you can stretch it as far as you want. But if there is no end point, you might feel awkward. So set your own end point. I call this the 'ten-shin (sky core).' In short, the center is body awareness of the straight line that connects the ten-shin and the chi-shin.

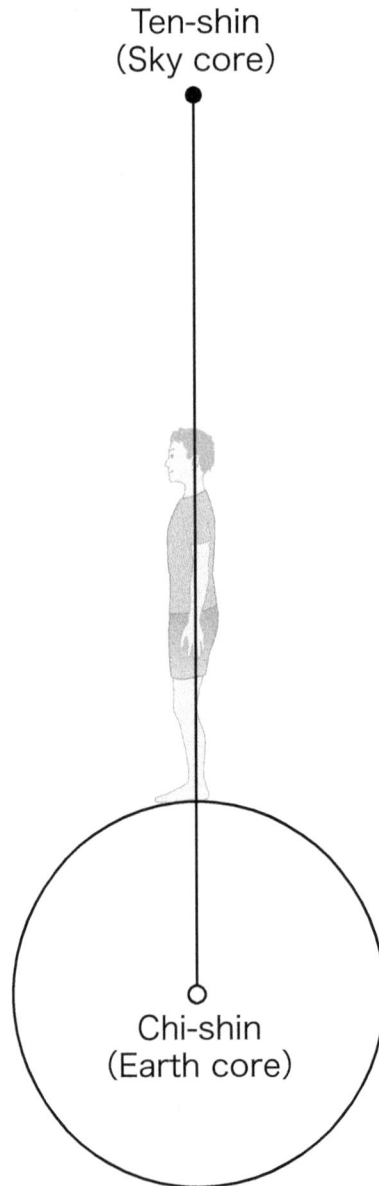

**The center is body awareness of the straight line
that connects the ten-shin and the chi-shin**

Ten-shin
(Sky core)

Chi-shin
(Earth core)

Body sense of the center

Now, let's discuss how you feel if you have the center in your body. First, you can stand straight. You have the sense of a higher center of gravity or a higher eye level. You might feel that your body became slender and taller.

The center works as a guideline and makes your knees and back straight. You do not need any extra energy to stand. It feels as if the top of your head is being pulled up by a string from above. This allows you to have a center axis in your body and rotate smoothly. Also, the balance of limbs improves. It makes your walking style smoother.

The center has a big impact on your mental side, too. Think about Michael Jordan. He is mentally stable. When he was active, he never got panicked but always acted calmly even under the enormous pressures or in critical situations he faced. He used to speak decisively and acted with a firm will. People with a well-defined center have such excellence. If your body does not require you to produce unnecessary extra power or if your body is nicely balanced because of the center, it will impact on your mind as well.

Also, if you have a stable core in your mind, you will no longer worry about small things. It doesn't mean that you will be insensitive. Because of your higher eye level, you can notice small things more acutely than a person who does not have a developed center. Yet you do not care about such small things. In other words, you can see things from a wider and higher point of view.

The center influences on human relationships significantly. It supports leadership. The most centered body awareness—that is a center. But I can of course say that, to be a successful leader, other body awareness types (the lower and middle tandens, the arch, the laser, etc.) are all needed, too.

The center and gravity line

Next, let's discuss what will happen in your body when the center is created. Here is a question for you. What is the big force acting on all objects on the earth including us human beings?

It is universal gravity − gravitational force. Gravity is a force that pulls objects toward the center of the earth. We are producing the same amount of power as the gravitational force by using our many muscles to keep standing, countering the force of gravity. The center is an awareness created by following the line that connects the center of gravity of an object and the center core of the earth. This means the center allows you to feel the positional relationship between your center of gravity and the center of the earth by maintaining perfect balance. It makes it possible for you to control your body's position in any posture. Therefore, the center can be called a high function device to create body balance.

The Iliopsoas muscles and the center

The center goes through between both sides of the Iliopsoas muscles. So what will the impact be to the body?

The iliopsoas is a muscle group that needs to be highly developed for any professional athletes to reach the top level. Have you ever heard 'the psoas major muscle exercise?' It is an exercise focused on developing the psoas major, which trims your waistline. The iliopsoas is the combination of the psoas major and iliacus muscles. I call it, especially the psoas major, 'the expert's muscle.' Why? Because of its location.

The psoas major is connected to two important parts; right underneath the hip joints that have the most important function in our body movements, and the lumbar and thoracic spine that is the center of the torso. The iliopsoas is connected to the center of the torso. It means it is located close to the center of gravity in the body. In other words, it controls the whole body from the point of the center of gravity. The center goes right in between the both sides of the psoas major.

The center goes between the iliopsoas muscles.

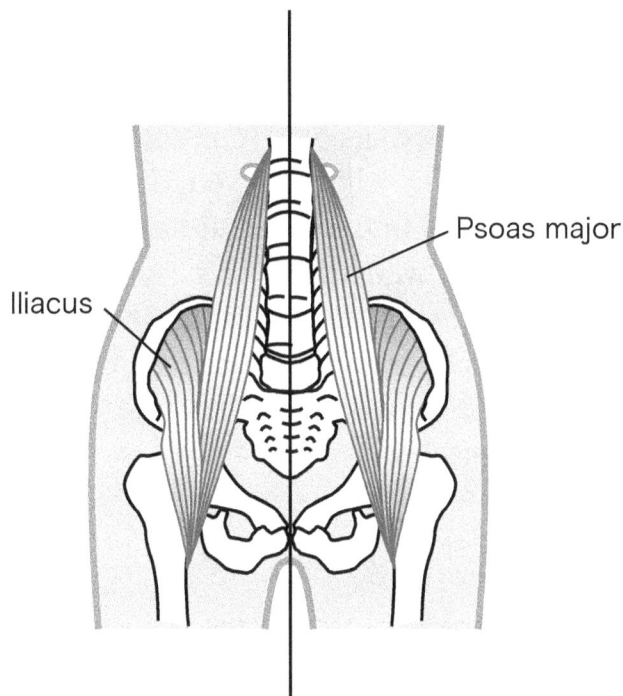

The iliopsoas muscles are the combination of the psoas major and iliacus muscles. The center activates the iliopsoas muscles, especially the psoas major, because it goes right between them.

As described in Chapter 1, body awareness stimulates activity of body parts where the awareness is working. Here is an experiment for you. First, think that you will start flexing your bicep in a couple of seconds. How do you feel in your arm now? Even though you have not produced power yet, don't you feel something in your arm? You might feel like your muscle starts moving.

Now flex your bicep.

Immediately before you flexed your bicep, didn't you feel strength in the area where you felt something during the above preparation? That is the body awareness. If you can create this awareness quickly and smoothly, you can produce power instantly. This is not surprising at all. When we focus on using muscular power at some location, certain awareness is always created there to prepare the muscles and bones at that location to get ready for a motion. If you do not focus awareness in advance, the muscles will not contract strongly. This means; if body awareness exists at a certain area, the muscles around that area always get ready and activated.

Let's get back to the story of the center. The center goes through the middle of the psoas major. It means the psoas major is always ready to work. If you learn to use the psoas major well, the position of your torso becomes aligned and your standing posture becomes nice and graceful. You can also walk smoothly. Furthermore, the position of your neck and the balance of your chin will improve as well as the balance of your facial muscles. This will make your facial expression more relaxed.

The fact is most super models in the world use their psoas major well - almost without exception. These models who have such beauty and poise and the top performing athletes who are active and starring in the sports world; they are exactly the same. They fully and capably use their psoas major muscles. The psoas major muscles are the secret of strength and beauty. The center is the body awareness that activates and controls those muscles.

Hamstrings and the center

The center also activates the hamstrings. The hamstrings are the muscles located on the backside of your thighs. They allow the fluid movement of the body of the super models or the super sprinting ability Rickey Henderson, who is widely regarded as the US major league's greatest leadoff hitter, used to show. (See the type 6, 'uratenshi (back push)' for more information about the hamstrings.)

Now, look at the locations of the hamstrings and the center. As you can understand from the previous experiment with your biceps, in order to activate the hamstring, it is ideal to have a well-developed awareness of such areas. That awareness is the sixth type 'uratenshi (back push).' The center is assisting the work of the uratenshi.

Look at the location of the center in the lower body. It is right in the middle of both sides of the uratenshi. You can use your hamstrings up to the maximum in the situation where the three lines, the center and both sides of uratenshi, are supporting each other.

The center activates the hamstrings

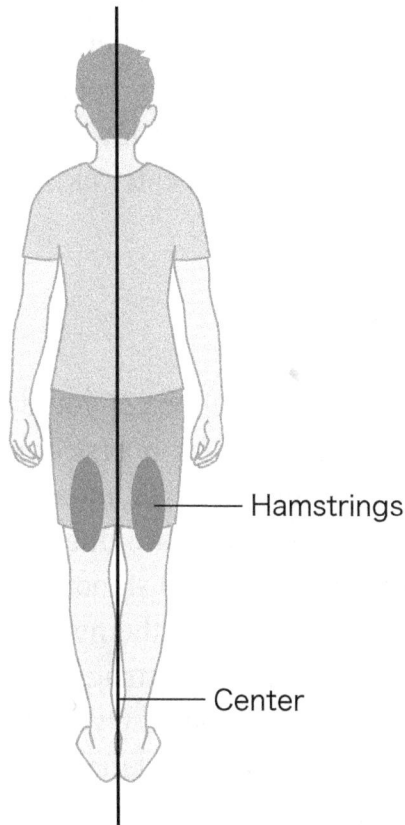

The sixth body awareness type, 'uratenshi,' is located on the hamstrings. Together with the uratenshi, the center activates the hamstrings.

Balance and the center

I have described the relationship between the center and the balance of the body. I am sure that you are already familiar with it. Next is the relationship between the center and each body part. It is like the string and pearls of a pearl necklace. Make a hole in the center of each pearl. Put a string through the holes in the pearls. Then, the scattered pearls become aligned on one line. No other method can be as accurate and easy to align the many pearls. The center works exactly like that. That is why Michael Jordan, Tiger Woods, and the super models that have the developed center can stand so gracefully using their center axis.

The center and the axis for rotating motion

What you must remember as one of the benefits of the center is it works as an axis for rotating motion. We can see many rotating motions in sports including swinging such as for baseball or golf. Even for walking, a pendulum motion of the limbs is required. So you must have the center axis. The center is taking the role of the axis and core in such movements.

Deficiency symptoms of the center

Here let's think about what will happen if you do not have a developed center. First, both your body and mind becomes overstrained. Each body part cannot be properly aligned without the center. However, most people have already gotten used to their bodies without the center. Therefore, they are not aware of the imbalance of their body parts. But how can they keep standing in such an imbalanced state?

That's because they are trying to firm themselves up by putting power into the whole body. Their knees are slightly bent, struggling to stay on their hips and feet, having too much strain in the neck or back, trying to hold on, pushing themselves too much, overstraining; these are the first deficiency symptoms of the center.

If you try to stay on your hips and feet while your knees are bent as well as your neck and back being strained, both your center of gravity and head are lowered. As a result, your eye level is lowered, too. This strained condition itself will affect your emotional feelings. Your field of vision and thoughts will get narrower. Furthermore, if you lack the center, you will more likely tend to overstrain and lose your mental balance, too. Both you and the people around you might believe that it is your personality. Wrong. It is actually because of the lack of the center. Most of the discomfort you are currently suffering from can be resolved just by developing the center correctly.

Then, what do you actually have to do?

You are trying to firm yourself up by putting power into your whole body. You are trying to prevent those body parts that are out of alignment from sagging or slumping. So, you need to release that power and loosen your body first. Then, you can create the center that is necessary to keep your balance. I will thoroughly discuss its training methods in Chapter 4. Here, I will just introduce you to a very good exercise called 'una tapping.'

Una tapping

As you can see in the illustration below, the lower legs have two bones, the tibia and fibula. The diameter of the fibula is only a forth or fifth of the tibia. It is obvious that the tibia is designed to support the whole body weight, but the fibula is not designed to do so. Despite that, most modern people put their weight on their fibula to stand and walk instead of using the tibia that is supposed to support their body weight, or some of them stand and walk while putting their weight on the front inner side of the tibia.

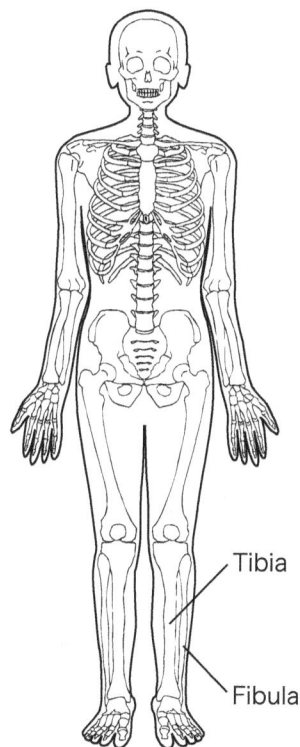

Tibia

Fibula

The diameter of the fibula is only a fourth or fifth of the tibia. Although humans are supposed to put their weight on the tibia when they are standing, many people put their weight on the fibula or stand in a position where the center of the tibia is misaligned to its front inner side.

So what happens to their body posture? If slanting to the fibula, their body weight is on the outsides (the small toe sides) of their feet and their knees are not touching each other. It makes them bow legged. On the other hand, slanting to the front inner side of the tibia makes them knock-kneed.

If your entire body is relaxed and has the center, you can put your weight on the center of your tibia. To stand like this, it is important to feel your soles right under the tibia. (It's on the inside of the arch of your foot, right under the ankles.) This point is called the 'una.'

If you create the una and put your weight on it, you can feel sensations such as "I am taller than usual," "I can stand easily," "I feel better," "I can see things around me better," or "I can breath easier." If you are very sensitive with awareness, you may feel like "Something like a line just shot through my body from the bottom to the top"—this directly describes how the center is developed. So if you have the body awareness of una, each part of your body gets aligned and it creates the center temporarily. But many people might think it is difficult to feel the una.

I would like you to try 'una tapping.' At first, determine the location of the una. Just like tapping on a shoulder, ask a friend to tap on your una 20 to 30 times to stimulate that part. You will feel a tingling sensation there and the body awareness is created. At last, just stand up while feeling the body awareness as a guide. You should be able to feel how to stand when the center is developed.

Una tapping

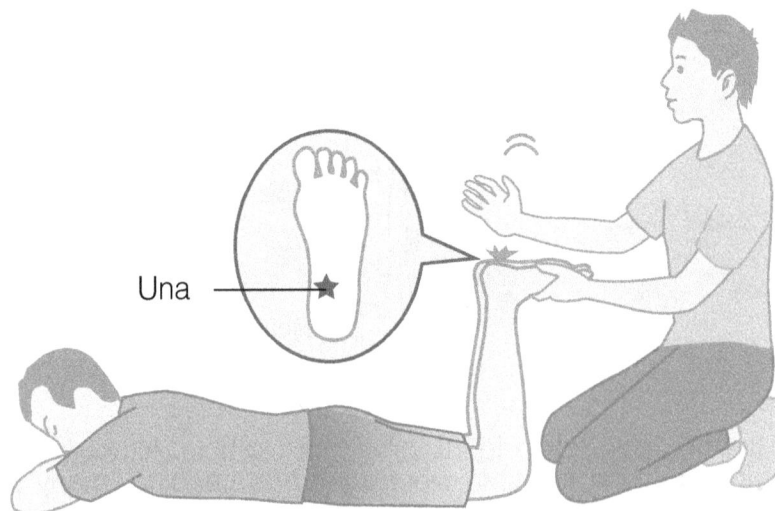

Una

Lie down on your stomach. Bend your knees 90°. Have somebody use the round edge of his palm, located on the heel of the wrist, and tap on your una 20 to 30 times to stimulate that part. (The una is on the inside of the arch of your foot, right under the ankles.) When you stand up, you will be aware of the una.

Type 2: Lower Tanden

For a long time, it has been said that the lower tanden is located in the middle of the lower abdomen, about 3.6 inches below the navel. This body awareness has been highly valued by Japanese people especially in the Edo period. Japanese samurai used to commit suicide by stabbing this area, an action called seppuku or hara-kiri.

For example, in order to convince or persuade an insane feudal lord, they committed hara-kiri to stop his unreasonable acts. This showed their honor and loyalty by giving their lives for their masters. Of course this custom cannot be said to be great. But why did the Japanese samurai commit hara-kiri? If the purpose were just to die, it would have been much easier for them to cut their carotid artery or stab themselves in the heart. But the samurai committed hara-kiri, because they believed they had the samurai spirit, the fundamental spirit to be a samurai, in their lower abdomen. This is the reason why the samurai killed themselves by cutting their abdomens where their core foundation exists.

Hara-kiri was supposed to be an honorable way to die, and quite different from "uchi-kubi" (decapitation) or "hari-tsuke" (crucifixion) which resulted from being arrested due to shameful charges. In other words, the samurai were permitted to commit hara-kiri only when their dignity was acknowledged. The location of hara (guts, intestinal fortitude) was the same as that of the lower tanden. Now, you can understand how much value the samurai families placed in the lower tanden in the Edo period that existed hundreds of years ago.

Today, the lower tanden is highly regarded in the world of Japanese traditional culture such as martial arts, Zen, Japanese traditional dance, Noh, or traditional music forms such as shamisen and shakuhachi. In these fields, the lower tanden is the key to improve respective performances.

I became able to feel the lower tanden when training for swordsmanship. What I felt was called 'dynamic tanden.' It is a very high level of the body awareness of the lower tanden. It has a high quality of mobility. It allows you to avoid sticking to the ground but to move freely and speedily while feeling the ground. You still feel like you are touching the ground firmly enough but simultaneously you are free from the ground.

This also works well for martial arts or sports such as aikido, sumo, judo that require scuffling. You can counter the other's offense using your lower tanden. If you can do it properly, the power of other's offence decreases by half. This does not mean you are still and just keep standing. You can move smoothly and quickly to a position for that is worse for your opponent to practice his/her offense.

The location of the lower tanden

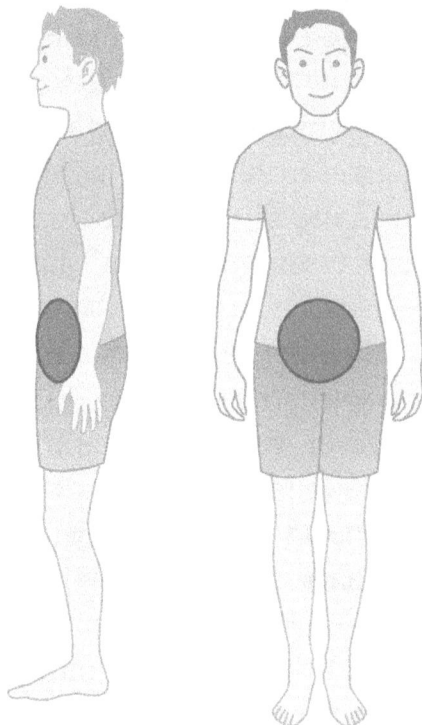

Body sense of the lower tanden

The body awareness of the lower tanden gives you a steady and unshakable mind. When you are mad or upset, don't you feel something hot is coming up in your body? You may feel an unsettled lower body and feel like your feet hardly touch the ground. The lower tanden prevents this kind of problem. Therefore, a person who has the highly developed lower tanden might seem to be too stable and difficult to approach by others. But in a situation when everybody is panicking, the person with the lower tanden becomes very important for the group.

Here is an example. A project team encountered and is stuck in a difficult problem. The members are exposed to many criticisms and are all disconcerted. But the team manager, who has the lower tanden, just tells them "Don't worry. It's ok to fail. I will take all responsibility." Then the team members can calm down and go back to what they are supposed to do.

The center gives you a cool clearheaded impression, higher eye level, and a more stable mind. You can see things from a higher and wider point of view. You will no longer be worried about small things. Then, what will happen to you when your lower tanden is developed?

You will not care about small things. But it is different from the situation that you see the things from a higher and wider point of view. It is more like the lower tanden pulls your upset feeling down from the bottom to keep you calm.

Also there is a difference in respiration. The center gives you bigger and vertically longer inhalations. But the lower tanden gives you deeper inhalations. In other words, the upper body becomes light and your breathing goes deeper down. This state is called 'jyou-kyo-ka-jitsu' in old Japanese. It literally means 'upper-empty-lower-filled.' The lower tanden typically creates this status in your body.

The lower tanden and the iliopsoas

Then why can you feel stable when the lower tanden is developed? This is closely related to how the body works. The lower tanden is located in the middle of the lower abdomen. More precisely, it is the body awareness created in between the navel and pubic joint. If you look at yourself from the side, the lower tanden is located slightly front of the center of the torso in the lower abdomen. If you have the awareness which has a heaviness sensation there, the iliopsoas is activated. This is different from the center. The center is a line that goes in between the psoas major muscles. The lower tanden is located more in front and is a globular shaped body awareness. That is why it especially activates the iliacus muscles.

The lower tanden and the diaphragm

Let's look at the lower tanden further. It is located below the diaphragm, the main respiration muscles. Thus the lower tanden activates not only the iliopsoas but also the diaphragm simultaneously.

The diaphragm is a muscle used for abdominal respiration. When the diaphragm contracts, it goes lower down. This expands the thoracic cavity and the amount of air in the lungs increases. When the diaphragm is relaxed, it goes up in a dome shape. This makes the air in the lungs decrease.

On the other hand, costal respiration requires the contraction and extension of the rib cage to force the air in and out. The volume of air coming into and going out from the lungs in one inhalation will be less than the abdominal respiration. This means the abdominal respiration is more efficient.

If you are able to do abdominal respiration well, the muscles around your chest will loosen because you do not need to overly use those muscles for breathing. Your shoulders will relax. You will feel calm and relaxed. Even if something upsetting happens, you can maintain normal breathing and continue to do the abdominal respiration as usual.

Respiration is a movement that you can control yourself, but also autonomic nerves control it. This means if you control your respiration well, you can control your autonomic nerves as well. Therefore even when a crisis or emergency occurs, if you can use your diaphragm well and keep performing abdominal respiration, you can face the challenge calmly and peacefully.

Recent biochemical studies have indicated that a hormone discharged from the bowels includes not only digestive fluids but also a component that has mentation activities. The lower tanden is the body awareness that is created in the area of bowels. It is not surprising that the lower tanden impacts a hormone discharge of the bowels that has circulatory impacts on the brain. So the lower tanden works for not just muscles and respiration but also directly works on the mental side through the brain.

The lower tanden activates the diaphragm

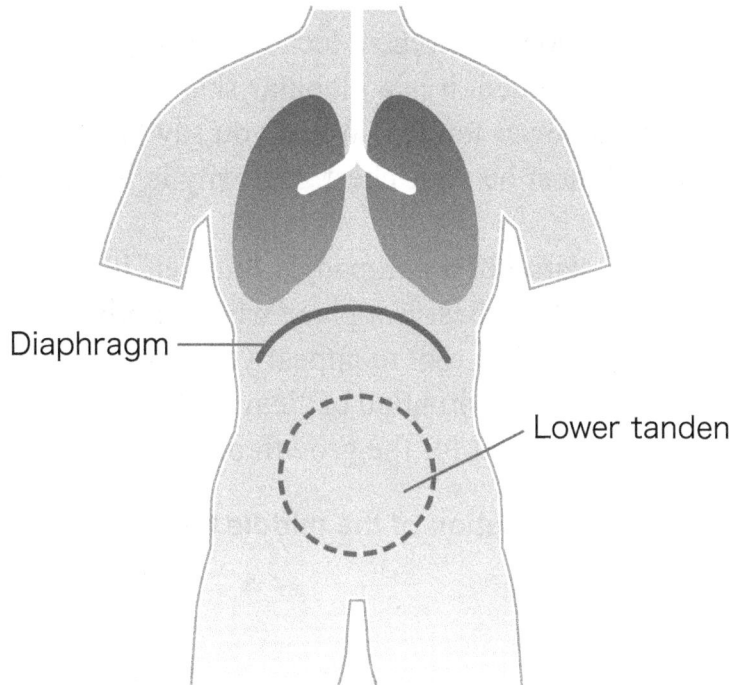

Diaphragm

Lower tanden

The lower tanden activates the diaphragm. When the diaphragm is activated, it is much easier to perform abdominal respiration. This produces a calmness and the volume of air coming into and going out of the lungs increases with each breath.

Deficiency symptoms of the lower tanden

If your lower tanden is weak, how will you be? First, you get upset easily. Your mind is restless and you do not feel at ease. Moreover, you run out of breath or find it hard to breathe. You may even be short tempered and get mad easily. It could make you go out of control with anger.

If you are like the above, you tend to think it is your personality and it cannot be fixed. Again, it is actually because of the lack of the lower tanden. If you have had this kind of problem for a long time, that means you tend to be upset for a long period and you would get mad often and easily. This could cause heart disease.

Type 3: Middle Tanden

The middle tanden is a body awareness located slightly below the center of your chest. Similar to the lower tanden, it is a globular shaped awareness but it tends to be slightly bigger than the lower tanden. When you say "leave it to me," where in your body do you tap? It must be your chest. But why is it the chest? Why not the belly, shoulder, or legs?

Imagine a picture or statue of a company's founder. It is most likely a sturdy upper body with chest out. The chest is a place where motivations like "leave it to me!" lives. It is also an expressive tool to appeal your motivation to others. That is why people tap their chests in the situation of "leave it to me!" The company founders swell their chests out to appeal for the growth of their companies.

The location of the middle tanden

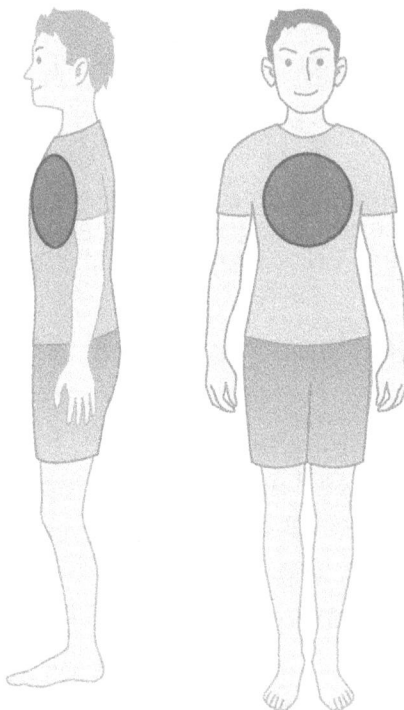

Body sense of middle tanden

If the middle tanden is created, you will be passionate. Your chest becomes warm and you can feel good excitement. You have a sensation of something being inflated. If the middle tanden works strongly, the sensation is something like boiling. This means the middle tanden is a body awareness connected to positive or aggressive actions.

For example, in sports, the middle tanden brings about fighting or gutsy performances. Gutsiness is brought about by the lower tanden as well. But the difference is the gutsiness brought by the lower tanden works as calmness or patience. In contrast, gutsiness from the middle tanden produces positive and aggressive actions.

In western culture, people say "a hearty person." This heart does not simply mean the heart as an organ. It expresses the heart as the center of emotion or passion itself. In this regard, I can say that the concepts of the heart and the middle tanden are similar. Cupid shoots his arrow into the chest, the area of the middle tanden. If you have passionate love, you have a strong middle tanden.

The middle tanden and heart function

Why is the middle tanden the center of motivation or passion? This has not been revealed completely. I haven't resolved everything. But I think it can be thought of like this.

Let's think about the location of the middle tanden. It arises in the area very close to your heart and the main arteries. If strong body awareness is developed here, the heart and arteries become activated. This sounds a bit technical, but when the middle tanden is created, two kinds of activations are happening simultaneously. Due to the action of the cerebral nervous system, your heart is activated and you can feel its activity clearly.

If you have the middle tanden, your heart, the blood stream around your heart, and the movement and the state of the blood vessels are all activated. At the same time you can actually feel it ten times more than a person who does not have the middle tanden. The heart is an organ that reacts very sensitively to the state of your mind. If you think about you are trying to do something, a command is sent through the cerebral nervous system, your heart becomes activated, and your heart rate increases.

If you do not have the middle tanden, you cannot feel anything even if your heart rate goes up. However if your body awareness is highly developed around the heart, you can unconsciously feel even just a few more heart beats strongly. In other words, you can catch the amplified stimulation of your heartbeat strongly at the subconscious level. If you feel your heart beat faster, you will feel it as a positive stimulation and become more excited and motivated. When this action operates in the brain, the motivated feeling produces another action that increases the heart beat. If this cycle repeats intensively, your heart rate keeps going up.

The middle tanden is linked to not only the heart but also the cerebral actions such as "I have to do something," "I have to move," or "I have to work." The heart rate and the emotion of "I will work," or "I will move" increase at the same time. This is why you can be motivated, energized and positive.

When the middle tanden activates the heart and the heart rate goes up, the sympathetic nerve is also activated as an inverse action. As a result, the hormone of the sympathetic nerve system discharges in the whole body. The sympathetic nerve will become predominant in the body. Therefore, if you have a highly developed middle tanden, you can show strong motivation both mentally and physically.

Now consider this. Who has a developed middle tanden among modern people? I would say Steve Jobs who passed away in 2011. In 2005, he gave an impressive commencement speech at Stanford University with the closing words "Stay Hungry. Stay Foolish." His middle tanden was truly burning. People who loved him, in other words, his fans, loved Job's energy and passion which came from his middle tanden. They wanted to get such energy from him. From the traditional Apple computer to the 21st century's products, iPod, iPad, and iPhone, his fans had been very impressed with his products as 'art' that are beyond simply devices. Job's middle tanden fired up his fans' middle tanden through the products.

Another typical person of the middle tanden was Bruce Lee, a Hong Kong film star who was famous for "Enter the Dragon." In the sports world, Babe Ruth, a US Major League baseball player, also had the developed middle tanden. The ski racer, Alberto Tomba, and the boxer, Muhammad Ali, both had the strong middle tanden as well. Outside of the sports world, the singer-songwriter, Lady Gaga, can be listed, too.

The middle tanden is kind of a source of explosive power. Someone who attracts people with such power can be categorized as a person with the middle tanden. However, too strong of a middle tanden has risks. If the middle tanden and lower tanden are well balanced, you can stay calm. But if your lower tanden is weak and your middle tanden is very strong, your sympathetic nerve rapidly increases because of the mutual action of the brain and heart. You cannot control your mind. When you train your middle tanden, you need to develop your lower tanden as well. It is important for you to practice to make the lower tanden control the middle tanden.

Deficiency symptoms of the middle tanden

Without the middle tanden, you don't feel motivated. You cannot love someone from your heart. You may like somebody but you cannot act like you love that person. In other words, you tend not to be passionate and motivated but rather gloomy and depressed.

The same thing applies to work, sports, and study. If at work, we wish to produce high performance and be successful. If in sports, we want to pursue great success and achievements. If in academics, we want to put our efforts focusing on our own subject and be confident in it. However, these motivations do not last long enough in many cases. Not just it. Some people may have a problem with a weak motivations or passions. This is a symptom of the deficiencies of the middle tanden.

Type 4: Arch

The arch is a body awareness creating an arched line that you make toward others or objects. It is also an awareness that you receive from others or feel their existence or emotions with your body and the center of your heart, and you respond to it appropriately in reverse. As you see in the illustration below, the line typically draws from or to your chest. But there is also a line of the arch coming from or to your head or back.

The shot of a basketball can be a good example of the arch toward an object. If you make a shot without aiming the ball carefully at the hoop, you are unlikely to succeed. However if you have the awareness between your hands and the center of the hoop before you make your shot, you will succeed easily.

For example, think about a shot by Michael Jordan in his prime. His shots used to go into the hoop as if a string pulled it. It is amazing that he could do it as quick as a flash from his shooting position. The string that pulls the ball is the arch. But it is not just about basketball. It applies to golf as well. Another example with which you are probably familiar is throwing something to somebody or throwing something into a trash box.

Using this concept, I have trained basketball players. Many of them showed higher success rates. One example involves the former captain of the all Japan team, Akira Rikukawa, who was called "Mr. Basketball" in Japan. He mastered the arch and won the title, "the king of the free throw," with the highest success rate ever in the Japan League.

The arch is not just for something you have toward objects. "He is very friendly even at the first meeting." "She seems to understand how I feel very well." Is there anybody around you about whom you feel so? Or is there anybody who you think has amazing insights into other people's subtle nuances or information? What they have is the fourth body awareness type, ' arch '.

Body sense of the arch

The first thing you have when you develop the arch toward people is a sense of connection. You can easily have a positive feeling toward others and tend to be friendly. It can be said that the arch is a body awareness that works for affinity. It creates a feeling that you are always thinking about them or you and others can understand well each other. Therefore you tend to enjoy going to places where other people are.

How can the arch be developed?

How can the arch bring you the body sense mentioned above? The secret is found in the early stages of the human development process. Think about the time when a baby starts to eat baby food. Parents let their baby sit on their laps or a baby chair and use a spoon to feed him. At such a time, do parents just hold out a spoon directly to a baby's mouth following a straight line? I don't think so.

Rather, the parents are likely to follow an arched line where even its curve is very slight and gentle. They talk warmly to the baby to prompt him to open his mouth. If you look at the movement of parents carefully, you will notice they first create the arched line awareness by moving their faces before they move their hands. Then, they feed the baby following that awareness line. It means the parents show an arched line awareness movement to their baby when he first learns how to receive an object from them.

Parents create the arched line awareness before they move their hands. They hand an object to the baby by following that awareness. What is this? This must be an expression of warm-heartedness. Parents have the feeling of warm-heartedness. That is why they hold out a spoon gently to their baby's mouth following a gentle arched line but not a sharp straight line.

Let's consider the baby's side. If the spoon is coming from his parents in an arched line, he can see and identify it without difficulty. If you actually test this, you can see the difference easily. An object coming to you following an arched line means that it goes up once and comes down. You would see the object much better than one coming to you directly in a straight horizontal line. This is the earliest example of development of the arch.

As the baby grows up, the parents and the baby start exchanging objects, like rolling a ball between the parents and the baby. Then they start tossing the ball rather than handing or rolling it. With the movements of the face and hands, the parents create the arched line awareness over and over again. Once they think the baby can recognize this line, they then toss the ball to the baby. The arch is developed and strengthened by such interactions and motions between the parents and their baby.

If you have a developed arch, you must have had many interactions at the early stage of development with people such as parents or grandparents who constantly and appropriately working on creating the arched line awareness towards you. Your arch has developed through such interactions. If you have the arch, you tend to feel like using it more unconsciously.

Where is your arch connected from your chest? It is basically connected to others. The arch itself is born from the feeling of 'warm-heartedness' intrinsically. That's why it reaches for other people's warm-heartedness. If you receive the arch from another, you will feel that person's warm-heartedness. At the same time, when you respond to it, you will feel like your warm-heartedness is revealed.

The development process of the arch

The arch is an arched awareness line coming in and going from your chest.

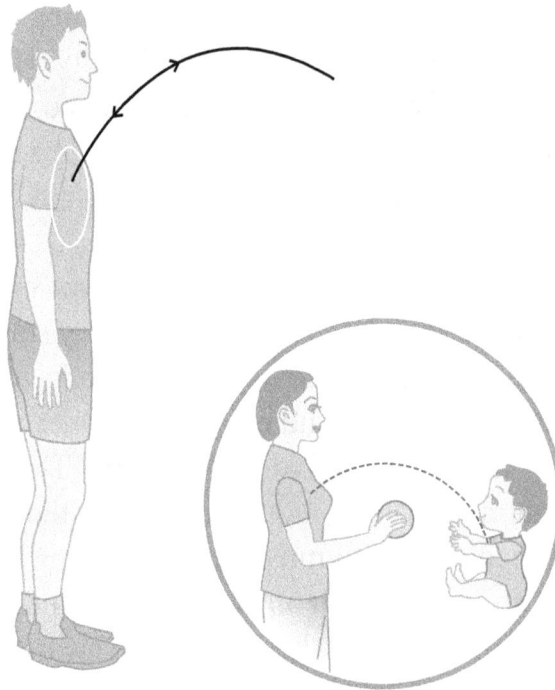

The arch is first created by the handing interaction between parents and a baby.

What happens when the arch is created?

Let's get back to the story of catch ball between the parents and the baby. With a good introduction by the parents, the baby can start throwing a ball back to the parents. However, the baby cannot throw well but keeps dropping the ball all the time at beginning. But the parents patiently show the baby how to do it using that line, their face, or hands. The parents who are good at teaching repeatedly tell the baby, "You can do it. You can use 'that'." in their subconscious mind.

'What is 'that'? Yes, 'that' is the arch. So the parents keep telling the baby subconsciously "That is it. The arch I created for you. You can use that thing." As a result, the baby develops the arch drawn from the parents' awareness. The baby can start having the arch toward the parents. It allows the baby to create the arch by himself and throw the ball back to the parents following an arched line but not a straight line. Then the parents give the baby much praise and say, "Wow, you are so good!" This makes the baby happy. The baby tries to use the arch more. When the baby becomes able to throw the ball back very well, the arch gets developed more and more.

The baby grows up into a person who receives the warm-heartedness from others but also who can give the same to others using the same awareness line. The arch allows us to receive the arch from others. Also, it allows us to give it to others. So there are two directions in the arch.

Thus if you have the arch and meet somebody, you will feel like treating that person gently without consciousness. You tend to say something gentle to him. The benefits and effects of the arch expand when you are grown up.

For example, there was a salesperson that was afraid of visiting his least favorite client. But, in front of the client's office, he created the arch by moving his hand and drawing an arched line from himself to the client's office. This action made him feel less afraid and brought him courage to open up to the client. When he met the client, the atmosphere was totally different from before. He could successfully and smoothly make business talk with them. This is a true story. I have heard many more stories like this from my workshop participants.

If you are shy about speaking in public, the arch is very useful. When you are waiting for your turn at the wing of the stage, you move your hands to draw the arch to connect it to various points in the audience. This will ease your tension and make you feel less nervous. But that isn't it exactly. You will have an affinity with the audience. When you stand on the stage, you will feel that you are welcomed by them. In such a situation, you never feel nervousness. Instead of nervousness or tension, you will feel empathy or pleasure.

Nervousness or stage fright can be controlled by the lower tanden, too. It works to stop you from being nervous or frightened but it doesn't work to create an affinity with the audience. In contrast, if you have a developed arch, you will not become nervous, but will have empathy. Thus, you can create great personal relationships with others.

Popularity and the arch

For professional athletes, musicians, politicians and so on who need to be popular, the arch is a must item. They have to attract people's hearts to be popular. Their arch has a close relationship with their popularity. Usually the arch works person-to-person. But for people like the stars, they connect the arch to hundreds or thousands of people at once. For national stars, they make the arch to millions of people. If it were a worldwide superstar's case, the number would be in the billons.

The arch cannot be developed at once. It is something developed gradually day by day while living as a star. However, the stars actually and originally had a higher arch than that of ordinary people. They brush up their arch more and more while climbing up to the stage superstardom.

So far, I have only described actors, actresses, or singers. In the case of the athletes, there are two types of superstars. For example, Ted Williams, a US major leaguer who had more than a 0.400 batting average, did not make the arch much. He was a typical center type person. His priority as a professional was the excellent play he could show to a crowd.

Even working in the same major league, Joe DiMaggio who played around the same time had a more developed arch than Ted Williams. He cared a lot for his US fans and the journalists. His sincere response and action to them was well regarded as an ideal baseball player. Ted Williams and Joe DiMaggio—they were completely opposite types each other, but they both were the excellent athletes.

Deficiency symptoms of the arch

The arch is a body awareness that works not just in one direction but also in the opposite direction. When you lack this awareness, you will first feel sad. You cannot be good with people. You cannot be friendly. Others cannot feel comfortable with you. Of course, you will never feel comfortable with them either. If those experiences are firmly set in your memory, you create this as part of your personality. It makes it harder for you to deal with people. This leads you to be isolated all the time or less confident about yourself.

In Japanese, 'human' reads as "ningen," which literally means "between humans." Humans are the creatures who need to associate with each other. We are creatures of communication. Our confidence is reflected by our abilities or skills. But also it is affected by how well we can communicate with people. Embracing human communication can be a big stress for you. 'Social withdrawal' of young people is one of the critical problems of today. It is also a representative symptom of the deficiency of the arch.

If you have the arch, you can control your anger and will not go ballistic. That is because the arch makes you have an affinity with others. When you tell something to others, both you and others feel a deep affinity to each other. Warm and gentle communications can be made. Your mind or intent can be conveyed to others straightforwardly.

In contrast, if you do not have the arch, you will feel that others do not understand how you feel. You will give up on them understanding you at all. You can only have a thin superficial relationship. As a result, your stress increases. You end up being unhappy. You cannot help hurting others.

Type 5: Vest

When you see top level people in various fields such as sports, martial arts, or calligraphy, etc., you will notice their usage of their upper bodies is way more flexible than that of ordinary people. The punching of Joe Frazier (a former champion of heavyweight boxing) and Rickson Gracie (a hero of Gracie Jiu-Jitsu), the swing of Tiger Woods; what is a common point for them?

When moving their arms, most people move them centering on their shoulder joints. However, how do the top level athletes move their arms? They are controlling their arms from the inside of their chest and back; deeper than their shoulder joints. There seems to be an awareness shaped like the arm holes of a vest. They move their arms as if these parts are also joints.

The fifth body awareness is called the vest. It is an awareness line on both sides. The lines go through several points; the middle of the collarbone, the breasts, the underarms, the point between shoulder blades and spine and come back to the middle of the collarbone. These lines very much look like the armholes in a vest.

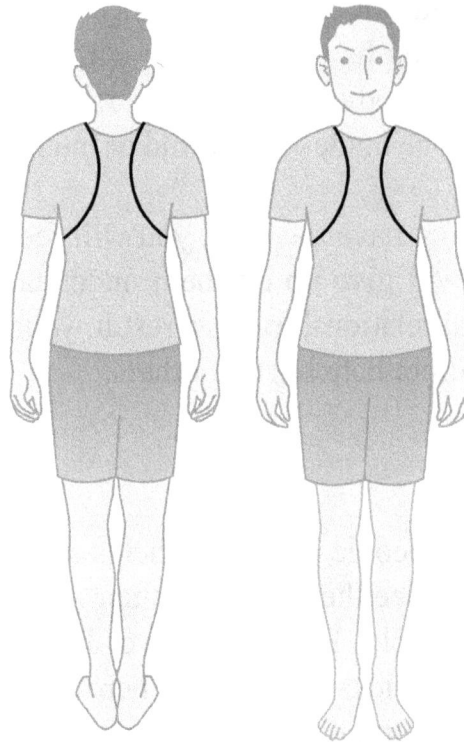

Body sense of the vest

The body awareness 'vest' allows your upper body to feel comfortable. You can use your arms in a good balance. To be specific, you can use your upper body well when playing any sports. You do not feel fatigue easily after carrying something. Your shoulders don't get stiff even after a prolonged period of typing. If you play a piano, you will find new techniques to play using the vest. If you are a cook, your knife cuts can be masterly.

There are benefits for hairdressers as well. Ordinary hairdressers move their whole bodies to changes their position to cut some difficult parts. But if you are a hairdresser who has the vest, you will easily move your scapular region to cut such parts. If you change the body position at each cut, the angle you look at the hairstyle always changes. Because this makes your image of the hairstyle change, too, the continuity of cutting can be broken. This is one of the reasons why some hairdressers can cut smoothly and freely but others cannot.

Now, you must have understood that the vest is that the body awareness which is beneficial if you are someone who requires good hands or arms movements. The vest also cures stiffness in your shoulders. Furthermore, the vest gives you mental benefits as well. If your shoulder area is relaxed and comfortable, you will feel a load off your mind.

The vest and the bones in the shoulder area

When I tell my students "move your arms back and forth," most people simply move their arms with their shoulder joints firmly fixed. Their ribs are stiff as a foundation and shoulder blades are like they are attached to the ribs and cannot move.

However, if you have the vest, you can move your arms more freely as if far inside of your shoulder joints, in other words, the lines of the 'vest' become big joints. Your ribs will be relaxed but not stiff. Your shoulder blades will be relaxed and you can use them freely. As a result, the flexibility around the base of the arms dramatically increases. The higher flexibility you have around the base or foundation of the arms, the easier you can move your arms.

If it is hard for you to imagine, think about a whip. The movement of your hand is expanded at the end of the whip. The same thing happens in your body. The movement of the base of your arms, even if it is a little movement, can become a big movement at your fingertips. This will reduce the workload of your shoulders and arms.

If your shoulders are fixed as a foundation, it will also impact badly on blood and other bodily fluids circulation. This creates the stiffness in your shoulder. The stiffness will not stop at the shoulders. You will have it in your back, underarms, and chest. It causes shallow inhalation and choking sensations - i.e., breathing difficulty.

Deficiency symptoms of the vest

If you lack the vest, you will have stiffness in your shoulders, back, underarms, chest, and throat. Unlike the rusty bicycle, you cannot be aware of your problem so easily. However, you will somehow feel like your upper body is stiff, that it's hard to breathe, and your shoulders feel unusually heavy.

'No vest' increases the burden on your arms or hands. You will feel fatigue in those parts. It can cause tendinitis. Even if it does not go that far, you will feel like avoiding any work in which you have to use your arms or hands a lot. Or you will feel annoyed or frustrated with such work. A large area of your brain is used to control the movements of your arms and hands which are burdened by the lack of the vest. You will have weariness and lack balance in your brain.

Nowadays, we are spending more time doing work that requires hand movements such as keyboard typing or texting. If you adjust and set your legs or torso according to the movement of your hands, or if you develop the vest and activate your shoulder blades, collarbones, and the many muscles around that area, you can have a good balance in your brain. However, if you only focus on your fingertips all the time, you will lose the balance of your brain and get tired easily.

Type 6: Uratenshi (Back Push)

The sixth body awareness type is 'uratenshi (back push)'. This is the strip-shaped awareness based on the area from the lower buttocks to upper hamstrings.

Body sense of the uratenshi

As mentioned in the section about the center, the uratenshi and the center help each other. Same as the center, the uratenshi also allows you to feel a high center of gravity. If you have the uratenshi, you will feel as if you are being supported by something from behind. I will discuss this more later, but I can guess that your front thighs, your quadriceps, must be developed enough and you are using them to support your body. However, if you had the uratenshi, you could support your body with a center focused on the area of your buttocks and back thighs. This means you are supported by something from the back side.

Imagine that you gently lean backward and rest your buttocks on a handrail behind you which is located at a slightly lower level. It becomes effortless to stand. If you have the uratenshi, you can always have this sensation. When you walk, you can easily step forward because you are supported and pushed from the back side. Some people feel exhilarated as if a nice comfortable breeze is blowing from the back to make them go forward easier or feel like they are being pushed by someone's big hands. There are also people who feel like they are being carried by a power from another dimension.

Walk, stand, climb up stairs, etc.; all these motions become easy to do. It impacts on your emotions as well. You will have less chances to feel "no, I don't want to do this," but easily go forward to start doing something.

The location of the uratenshi

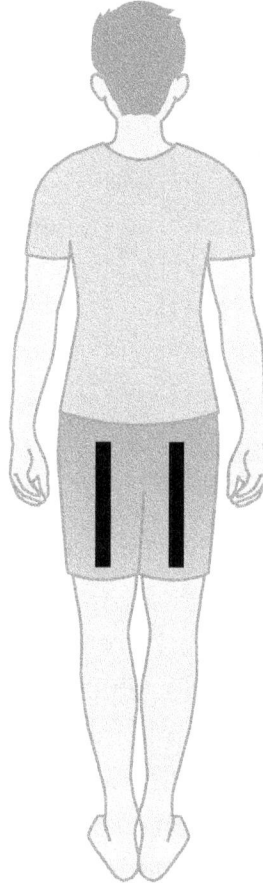

The uratenshi and the hamstrings

Look at the illustration below. The quadriceps are located in the front side of your thigh. And the hamstring is located in the back side of your thigh. For example, the star players of the World Cup soccer teams have a more developed awareness of their hamstrings than that of their quadriceps. Why can more excellent movements be performed by using the back side of the thighs than the front side?

Quadriceps —

Hamstrings

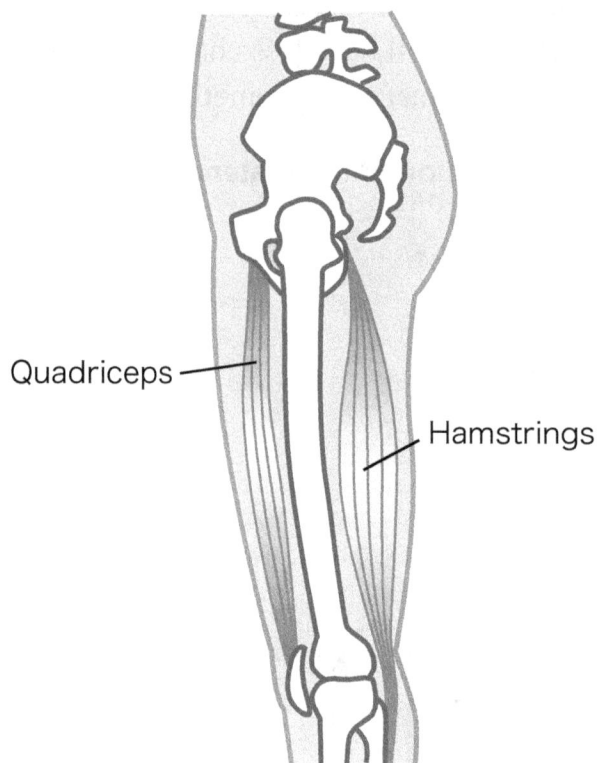

Think about walking down a hill. If you walk normally, you naturally speed up and it is difficult for you to stop. So what happens to your body then? You are unconsciously making a resistance step by step using your front thigh muscles not to speed up and lean forward. That's why, after you walked all the way down, you will notice your front thighs have gotten really hard.

You can also think about stopping suddenly while you are dashing at full speed. You will make as much as possible resistance using the front thigh muscles. The front thigh muscles, quadriceps, have a role as the brake to resists the attempt to move forward. Then, if you can use your hamstrings, what will happen?

When the hamstrings are activated around the hip joints, in other words, when they contract, the thighbones swiftly swing backwards just like a windshield wiper with the center being the hip joints. That movement is transmitted to the ground. As a reaction, it produces the power to lift up and accelerate the body diagonally forward. Therefore you can move forward with a high center of gravity.

If the body awareness, uratenshi, is created on the hamstrings, do you know what will happen? Yes, the hamstrings become activated.

Let's get back to the story of the top-level soccer players. As their hamstrings are very developed, they can often keep playing the game even if they hurt their quadriceps by running into other players.

By contrast, players who have not completely reached the top-level cannot continuously play, not even practice, if they hurt their quadriceps. What does this mean? It means that although the world's top players and ordinary players look almost the same from the viewpoint of running or kicking the ball, the muscles they use are totally opposite. For example, most Japanese players tend to use their quadriceps more. However, some recent players such as Keisuke Honda, Shinji Kagawa, or Yuto Nagatomo have started to use their hamstrings more than their quadriceps.

Early people had a high developed uratenshi

As explained above, the hamstrings work to swing thighbones backward with a center on the hip joints; it is part of the process of moving your body forward. That is why I call these hamstrings 'accelerator' muscles. When the hamstrings are working well, it produces excellent movements.

In an earlier age, people lived by hunting. They hunted animals to survive. To make this possible, they were required to make overwhelmingly quick movements on a daily basis. They must have fully used their hamstrings as 'accelerator muscles.' When they travelled far for hunting, they also needed quick movements to escape from the possible danger of being attacked by beasts.

If moving quickly or fast produced good results, how do you think humans should feel about the body usages that provide you with such good results? Comfort or discomfort? The brain should have recognized that it was comfort. If we human beings feel discomfort with the movement which creates good results, we would have become extinct.

With the developed uratenshi and the activated upper hamstrings which are close to the hip joints, anybody can feel nice and comfortable. I am sure that this relationship has been incorporated into our DNA. This concept is part of 'kinetic evolution theory'. Human beings could not survive unless we kept seeking for rationality in the history of evolution. It is very interesting that such reasons and results can be seen when looking back at the various stages of human evolution.

Deficiency symptoms of the uratenshi

When you lack the uratenshi, you first feel too lazy to walk. Even if you try to walk or go somewhere, you will put a brake on yourself subconsciously. Therefore when you actually start walking, you have to force yourself to go forward and release the brake on your mind.

On the other hand, if you have the uratenshi, you can feel like you are walking down a low-pitched slope even if you are on a flat surface. You can smoothly step forward without any hesitation. Even if you could use a bus or train, you don't feel lazy about walking all the way to the next stop. You can easily accept and enjoy work that usually makes you feel annoyed. This greatly reflects on your mind. It makes you act positively.

The third body awareness type, middle tanden, brings you positiveness as well. But this is more like the positiveness related to aggressiveness due to the action of the sympathetic nerve system. The uratenshi allows you to go forward spontaneously.

If you are a business person and have the uratenshi, you will notice yourself motivated and acting forward all the time. But if your uratenshi is not fully developed, you would be hesitant to do anything and become inactive. It is because you are putting a brake on yourself subconsciously. So you have to try to motivate and convince yourself before taking an action. You are consuming a lot of mental effort and energy unnecessarily. It is like there is a hurdle placed just in front of you.

Type 7: Laser

The last body awareness type is called 'laser.' The fourth type of 'arch' is an arched line. But as you can see in the illustrations below, the laser is a straight horizontal line toward others or other things.

Laser and aim

In martial arts, sports, performing arts; all movements require physical orientation and transferring motion. These fundamental elements are closely related to the laser. In Chapter 1, I explained that you cannot walk well unless you have the awareness of two lines vertically and horizontally. The vertical line is the center that I have already discussed. The laser is the horizontal line that I want to describe now.

I will give you another example of the bicycle. Some people ride on a bicycle very well, but others don't. People who are good at riding can smoothly keep finding open spaces to ride and can stop quickly without effort. On the other hand, people who are not so good seem to be wobbly and almost fall down.

What makes this difference? When you are trying to start riding a bicycle, is there anything that works in a traveling direction? You must have an awareness in front of you at a subconscious level which is a straight horizontal line aiming you in one direction. Using that guideline, you can start riding smoothly toward your destination. The difference between a good cyclist and a bad cyclist is related to the strength of this body awareness. In other words, there are two different types of people; those who can create the awareness strongly and those who cannot.

Next, let's think about sports. For example, track and field: Like Usain Bolt or Tyson Gay, all track and field athletes have a developed laser. Without an extremely strong awareness aimed at their goal in the 100 meters, they could not be star athletes in their fields. Maurice Greene who previously attracted people's attention also has the developed laser.

Swimming is supported by the laser as well. As you might have experienced, the more you use your full energy, the harder for you to swim straight. There must be many people who have almost hit a lane rope when swimming really hard. However, top-level swimmers, such as Michael Phelps, can swim very straight without wandering from side to side. It can be said that they can do it because they are swimming led by a highly developed laser.

Tiger Woods has the developed laser as well. First, he aims for the target extremely straight. Next, he determines the ball line to the cup. That is a laser. Then, the arch of the up-and-down movement of the ball is added on the laser. At last, he controls his body movement (swing) by following back on that line.

The laser and the sacrum

The basic type of the laser at a standing pose is a line of the awareness that stretches straight forward from the center of the sacrum. Why does the laser need to be stretched from the sacrum? The reason is because the sacrum is the bone that supports the head, arms, and torso.

Sacrum

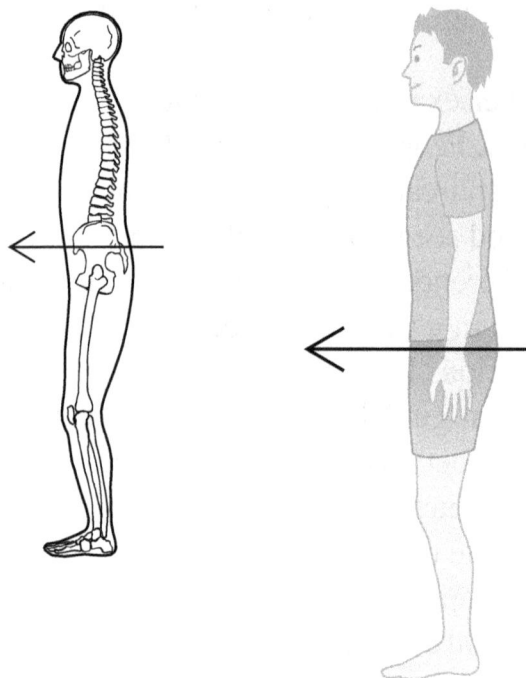

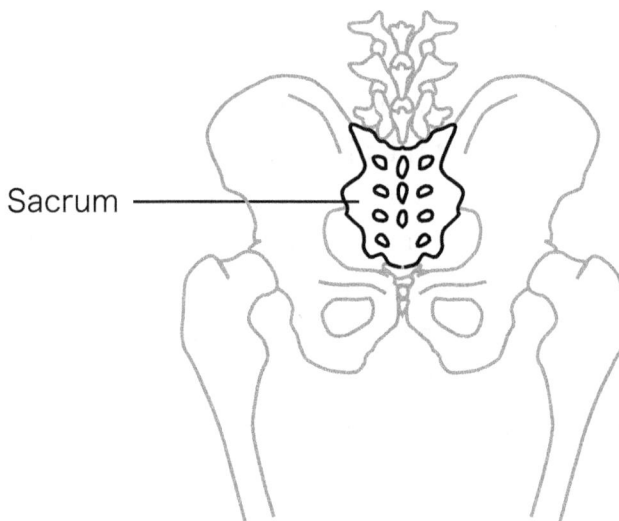

Think about the history of evolution. Humans are a vertebrate animal. Vertebrate animals started with fish. The vertebrate was fully developed in the era of fish. However, fish do not have the sacrum. The reptiles that evolved later and live on the ground have no sacrum either. Nor do further evolved creatures such as mammals with four legs have the sacrum as strongly as humans.

So the full-blown sacrum is a bone unique to us humans. When you look at the sacrum carefully, you will notice it is fused with five sacral vertebras to make one bone. It means that if humans were animals of the old age, the five sacral vertebras would be separately aligned. But as a human bone, all five sacral vertebras were fused and have become wider.

By looking at the history of the human evolution as well, it is no doubt that the sacrum was developed and designed to support the upper body for walking upright and supported by two legs. In this sense, it can be said that the sacrum is one of the very important parts of our bodies.

Also, the sacrum is located in between the hip joints. The cervical spine, thoracic spine, lumbar spine; all the spines except the coccyx are on the sacrum. The hip joints that work as an axis for rotating legs are located evenly side by side of the sacrum. It means the sacrum is not just the center of the upper body but also the center of the lower body.

From this point of view, the sacrum is located in the perfect position as a starting point of the laser that is the guideline for a human to walk or run. If you have the laser in the middle of the hip joints that are the two rotating axes to swing the legs, and use it as a guideline to move forward, it will be easy for you to control such an axis.

The whole upper body is located on these two axes. The hip joints have to work as a rotating axis while carrying the heavy upper body. If you have the laser in the area where the upper body weight is on, you can use it as a device to maintain balance. Simultaneously working a great amount to keep the body balanced, the laser works to adjust and maintain the balance of the rotating axis of the thighbones to support and carry the upper body.

The laser and the aiming function

Imagine you are exchanging something with somebody. As contrasted with the arch, the laser is used to throw something straight like an arrow. It creates a rather adversarial relationship with others. A very tense relationship as if an arrow is driven between you and others will be produced.

Parents use the arched line, the arch, to give and take the warmth and caring. On the other hand, when siblings are fighting and throw something at each other, they use the laser to throw it hard with hostility.

When thinking back to ancient times, probably everyone used to live by hunting. The movements of throwing stones or sticks to kill their prey had been made repeatedly for a long time. To get the prey, it is important to have the skill to throw or act accurately. The laser must have been developed as an aim for that. (This is an applied type of the laser that starts from the chest, but fundamentally supported by the basic laser starting from the sacrum.)

Therefore, the athletes who require throwing a ball have a highly developed laser. Excellent US Major League pitchers are definitely some of them. For example, the fast sharp throwing of Nolan Ryan or Roger Clemens can evoke a laser beam.

On the other hand, another Major League player, Babe Ruth, is a typical arch type. He had an remarkable arch and his home run ball followed an especially high arched line. It is totally opposite compared to the batted ball of Ichiro who has an incredibly developed laser which goes lower, sharper, and straight.

Body sense of the laser

I explained that the laser brings out strong tension. In our daily or business lives, having the laser can be beneficial to you. As described above, you can use the laser as a guideline to reach the goal and aim at your target. If you have the developed laser, you can act coherently to reach your goal or accomplish your target.

For example, if you are a businessperson attending a meeting, you can quickly point out necessary issues. When the discussion goes off on a tangent, you can always pull it back to the right course. But this type of person may look too sharp and a bit unfriendly.

A person who has the arch is opposite. The arch type person begins a meeting by creating affiliation with others. As a result, others feel comfortable in a warm atmosphere. Everyone has a feeling of wishing to help one another. So they can create and exchange many good ideas.

It is best to have both the laser and the arch. You won't have any problem with having these two together. There are no contradictions. All of the seven body awareness types that I have discussed work to help each other. Having multiple awareness types never brings you any negative effects. It is good to have one body awareness type. It would be better to have two awareness types. If you have three or four of them, you will get even more benefits both mentally and physically. Athletes, artists, business professionals, doctors, teachers; in any fields, successful people have many body awareness types. The more excellent people are, the more body awareness types they have.

Special column: Heel line

Other than the seven body awareness types, there is another wonderful awareness called 'heel line.' The heel line is an awareness created from the heels.

You might think that the calf, Achilles tendon, heel, and foot make the letter L and the heel is a corner of its right angle. This is wrong. The heels have calcaneal bones sticking out from underneath the talus, the ankle bones, that are right below the tibia. So it is shaped more like the upside down letter T rather than the L. If you are not aware of that, you cannot use those ankle bones. Many people might think you can move quicker using tiptoes. This is completely wrong. In fact, all the experts, regardless of era or cultures, walk using their heels. "Stand with tiptoes" is the opinion of people who have not reached the experts' level.

The location of the heel line

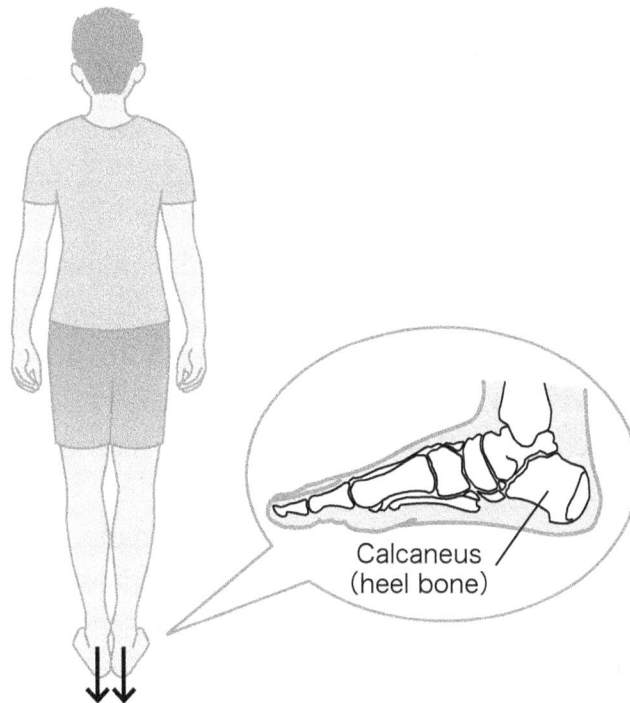

Calcaneus
(heel bone)

Using the calcaneus well produces strong starting power.

I have mentioned Ichiro many times in this book as a representative of people who have a highly efficient body. He is a typical expert who uses his heels. He is well known for his base stealing. He uses his heels very well. The body awareness, the heel line, that stretch down from the heels, can produce such a movement. Ichiro's seamless dashing after getting a hit, and his base stealing techniques; they are all achieved by the heel line.

Actually, if you compare his highest running speed with that of other players, he is only average among Major League players. However, his excellent starting dash is among the fastest of current players. When carefully watching Ichiro's dash, his heels are fully touching the ground and he puts his weight on them for the first, second, and even second and a half steps.

Usually many people think that it is more effective to dig into the ground with their toes. So their heels immediately hover from the first step. However, Ichiro tends to keep his heels touching on the ground and his heel bones pushing on it as long as possible. Also, Rickey Henderson was a great Major League player who was called the "Man of Steal." I repeatedly saw his video. His heels, too, firmly touched the ground and his heel bones pushed it for the first four steps when dashing.

If you produce a propulsive force with your heels, you can deeply and powerfully move your body forward. It is hard to see but a tremendous power is hidden in 'the heel line'. The successful athletes whose starting dash is very important always have the heel line. For example, sumo or judo do not require many steps in a game. But the heel line makes a great impact when starting off or receiving a push from opponent and pushing it back.

I mentioned that the heel line has been an important awareness among all experts regardless era or cultures. In Japan, there is a textbook called "Gorin no Sho (The Book of Five Rings)" written by Musashi Miyamoto, one of the most famous Japanese samurai. It is written about kenjutsu (technique of the sword) and martial arts in general which is considered the greatest classic treatise on military strategy.

In the chapter of Water, there is a section on "Footwork." In this section, Musashi wrote "With the tips of your toes slightly hovering, tread firmly with your heels." For a long time, this method had been hard to understand by many researchers who studied Musashi and The Book of Five Rings. Because in today's martial arts' world as well as in the sports world, it is more common to think like "grab the ground with your toes" or "hover your heels only for the space of a piece of paper."

However, since I was young, I have understood from my experiences as a martial artist that it is very important to use the heels to push on the ground and not stand on tiptoes to push down when making strong and quick movements. So when reading The Book of Five Rings, I was fully convinced by Musashi's words and thought "Musashi also knew how important the pushing down with the heels was."

If the heel line is developed, you can make a quick and strong first step. When you try to move something inert, you need a power greater than the force of its inertia. In a lowest velocity state that requires a strong force to start moving, the power produced by the heel line will be extremely effective. This is similar to a low gear of a car. Once moving, speed would be more important than strength just like in a car where you would naturally shift up from a lower gear to a higher one. So, kicking on the ground with the toes becomes effective. But before then, the deep strength from the heel line would work and mean a lot.

As you develop the heel line and it influences not only on your physical movements but also your actions, you will no longer feel too lazy to do something, even a small starting movement required in your daily life or at work. You will feel energized from deep in your body. You can start moving effortlessly. You will not need to try hard to motivate or convince yourself to do something.

Chapter 3

Body Awareness Check Test
Which body awareness type best describes you?

Why can't you use your body efficiently and effectively?

After you have read this far in the book, you might be interested in how much body awareness you actually have. At the same time you may be wondering how it can be determined. In fact, you can determine with a relatively simple test if you have body awareness or which awareness is strong or weak. In this chapter, I introduce to you 'the body awareness check test.' Take this test and find your body awareness level.

In this test, there are five statements for each of the seven body awareness types. Most statements address your personality or action patterns. For example, "I don't get disturbed in any circumstance," or "I often go off the track and cannot achieve my goals." Also there are statements that address your feelings or actual body sensations, such as "When seeing myself in a photo, it looks like there is an imaginary straight line that goes up and down through the center of my body."

Some readers may wonder why there are no statements about athletic abilities like "I can throw a ball very far," or "I can hit a ball accurately." These abilities depend on what kind of sports you do or how much experience you have in sports such as baseball or golf. Even with a developed vest, if you have never played catch, you would not be able to throw a ball well. Similarly, even with a developed center and laser, if you have no experience playing golf, you would not be able to hit a ball accurately.

Therefore, the statements here are unrelated to your athletic experience. All statements apply to all readers to allow you to answer and judge yourself easily. Be honest and natural. Discover the body awareness that you have. Enjoy!

The Seven Body Awareness Types Check Test

What is missing in your body and mind?

Before you take this test

There are three ways to use this check test for evaluating your body awareness. Please refer to the notes below:

(1) Measure yourself to learn which body awareness types are developed or lacking.

The check test helps you notice which body awareness types are developed and those that are actually lacking in your body. The important thing is to be as honest and natural as possible. If you answer with hope or assumptions, your test results may not be reliable.

Please note that the results that are made in this way are subjective. If others evaluate you using this check test, their results will be objective. Your results and their results about you will be different. Simply comparing those two results is not recommended.

(2) Keep practicing the body awareness training and regularly measure yourself to know what changes or achievements can be seen.

Taking the test regularly (once a month or so) helps better understanding of how you are changing yourself. If you get used to this test, the reliability of your evaluation will increase. This is the most appropriate use of this test for you to understand the theory of the body awareness and master its training methods.

(3) Regularly take the test with your friends or family to evaluate yourself and each other, to compare such results, and to improve your evaluation technique.

Taking the test with your close friends or family is helpful. Be honest and stay unemotional. Compare with all results and discuss the appropriateness of your and their evaluations. If you take the average of such evaluation results, you can expect to see your body awareness more objectively and accurately.

Important notes

This check test is not the most appropriate way to evaluate top athletes or celebrities like those who are featured in this book. In order to compare two or more top-level people accurately, more technical and specialized methods are required. I have used such methods and an expert approach to study the body awareness of those people in this book. Therefore if you evaluate a top athlete or celebrity simply based on the information from media, the results can be used as a general guide, but will not be very reliable.

Directions:

There are five statements for each test of body awareness. The numbers 1 to 5 describe the level of how much it applies to you. Your task is to indicate the strength of your agreement with each statement using the scale below. 1 denotes strong disagreement, while 5 denotes strong agreement. And 2, 3, and 4 represent intermediate judgments. Enter a number from 1 to 5 for each statement and write down the total score under the statements for each type of awareness.

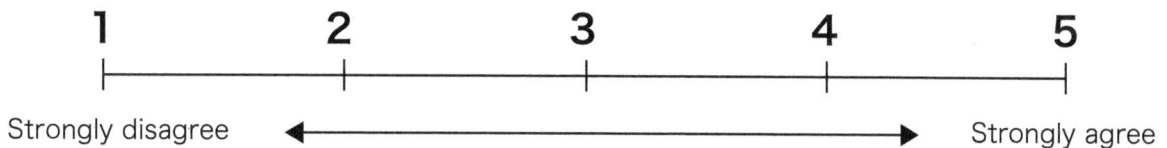

```
    1           2           3           4           5
    |-----------|-----------|-----------|-----------|
Strongly disagree    <------------------------>    Strongly agree
```

Test 1: Center

1) I can act as a leader or center of a group. (   )
2) I see things from a wider and higher point of view. (   )
3) I can always feel breezy and clear in my mind and have a similar body sensation. (   )
4) When seeing myself in a photo, it looks like there is an imaginary straight line that goes up and down through the center of my body. (   )
5) My way to live, think, and talk is coherent and has a stable core. (   )

Total = (   ) points

Test 2: Lower Tanden

1) I feel a robust sensation in my abdomen and hips. (   )
2) My actions, behavior, or thoughts are firm and steady. (   )
3) Others can rely on me in a pinch. (   )
4) I do not get mad or upset in any situation. (   )
5) I can breathe deeply and stay calm in a situation where mostpeople would be disturbed. (   )

Total = (   ) points

Test 3: Middle Tanden

1) I am very energetic. (   )
2) I can love somebody passionately. (   )
3) I often feel impressed, touched, or excited by something. (   )
4) When the need arises, I feel "you can rely on me." (   )
5) When seeing myself in a photo, I feel the force of my confidence from the chest. (   )

Total = (   ) points

Test 4: Arch

1) I like speaking in front of many people. (   )
2) I can easily get along even with a person who looks unfriendly. (   )
3) I am good at working or doing something with others. (   )
4) I like people and I tend to be liked by others. (   )
5) I am good at asking somebody to do something or joining in other's conversations without ruining the atmosphere. (   )

Total = (   ) points

Test 5: Vest

1) I have a relaxed informal image. (   )
2) I feel in control and breath normally even in a situation where most people feel uncomfortable and their shoulders get stiff. (   )
3) I am good at doing light work that requires the use of my arms such as dishwashing, cleaning a table or windows, wiping things, or organizing books. (   )
4) When seeing myself in a photo, my shoulders look very relaxed. (   )
5) Even when I am busy and have many things to do, I can keep working without feeling stiffness in my neck or shoulders. (   )

Total = (   ) points

Test 6: Uratenshi (Back Push)

1) When standing, I feel a high center of gravity. I stand straight and disciplined. (I do not sag nor hold on to things.) (   )
2) I walk gracefully without bending my knees and lowering my hips when I put my foot down on the ground. (   )
3) I can walk smoothly and comfortably. I even feel my body as it moves forward naturally and effortlessly. (   )
4) When walking up a hill or stairs while carrying something heavy (ex. when moving house), I often feel that I am using the back of my thighs rather than the front. (   )
5) I can easily move or act forward even if there is resistance oran obstacle. (   )

Total = (   ) points

Test 7: Laser

1) People have said to me or I think that my gaze is strong and sharp. (　)
2) I can find a target (thing or person) in a crowd quickly. (　)
3) I can go straight toward a goal that I determined as if the goal and I are connected with a straight line. (　)
4) I can point out issues accurately or adequately. (　)
5) I can walk smoothly and quickly even in a crowd. (　)

Total = (　) points

1. Check your score against the following grading scale.

25   S = Superior
20-24   A = Very good
15-19   B = Good
10-14   C = Fair
5-9   D = Deficient

2. Write your results in the table.

	D 5~9	C 10~14	B 15~19	A 20~24	S 25
Center					
Lower Tanden					
Middle Tanden					
Arch					
Vest					
Uratenshi (Back Push)					
Laser					

3. Create your radar chart.

Mark the point for your score for each awareness type then connect all points.

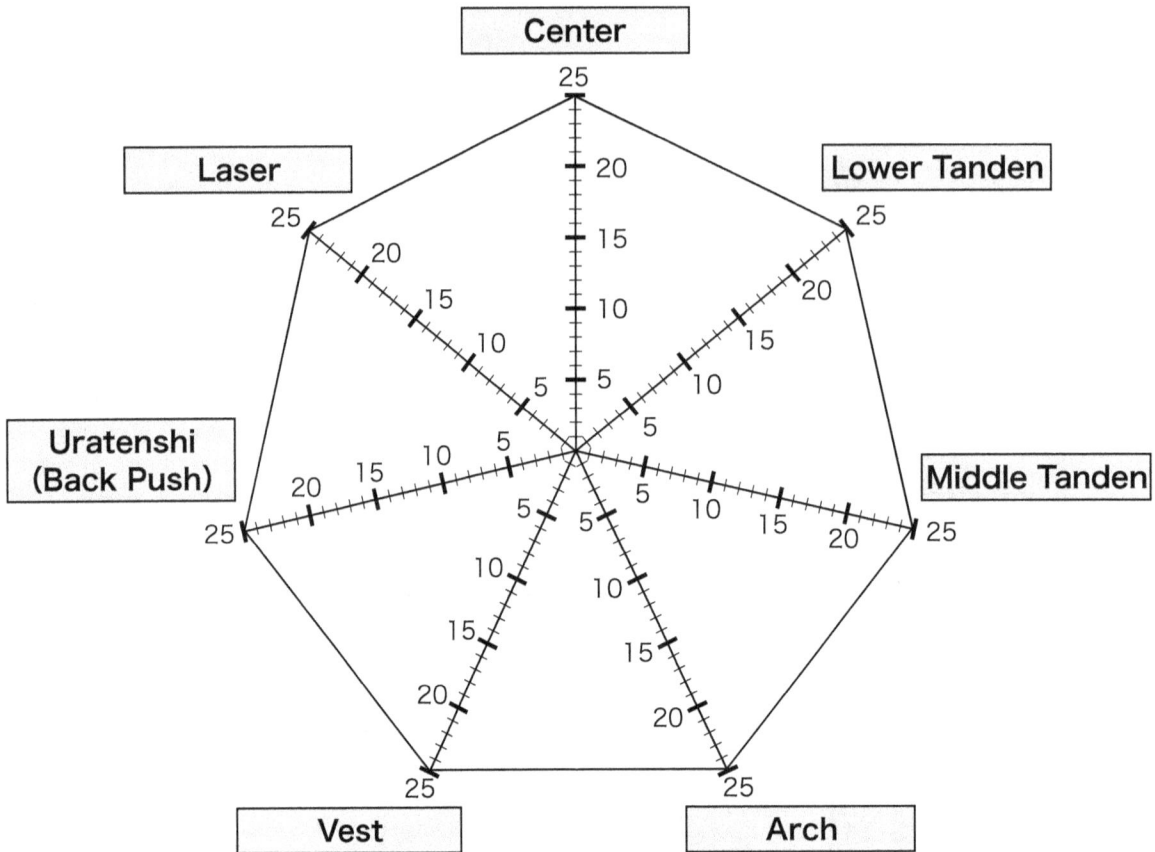

Evaluate your test result

When you are done with the test, add up your total score for each body awareness type and put your results in the above table. How does it look?

I have a sample result here. Let me explain how to read the table and chart using this sample.

	D 5~9	C 10~14	B 15~19	A 20~24	S 25
Center			15		
Lower Tanden		14			
Middle Tanden			17		
Arch			17		
Vest		14			
Uratenshi (Back Push)			15		
Laser				20	

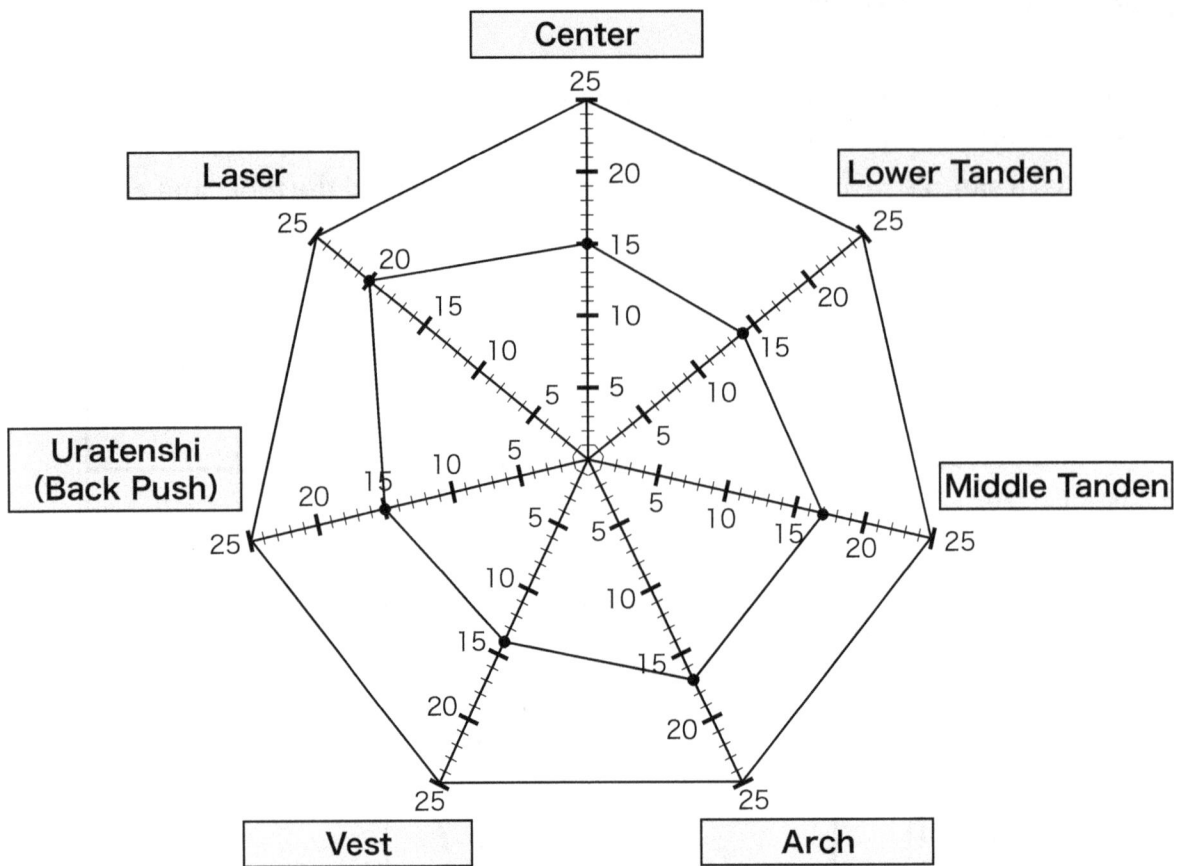

This sample shows the test results of a sportswriter I know. His center is 15 points; that is the score B. His lower tanden is C, both the middle tanden and the arch are B, the vest is C, the uratenshi is B, and the last item, the laser, is 20 points, A. He is most developed in his laser. Then his middle tanden and arch follow. From these results, I can tell that he is a person who is passionate and good at dealing with people. Also that he tends to set his goals and successfully reaches them.

As for his center, lower tanden, vest, and uratenshi which all scored B or C, there is room for further growth. If he develops more in these areas, he will be able to exert higher performances both privately and officially. He should focus especially on his vest that will allow him to use his back and chest areas more flexibly. While maintaining the sharpness from his laser, the vest will allow him to soften his harshness. He should be able to develop more constructive relationships with others.

Similar to this, if you look at your score for each body awareness type, you can see the tendency of your actions, behaviors, or thoughts. To see such tendencies more clearly, use the radar chart. Mark the point for your score in each awareness type then connect all points. You can see your character (tendencies) as a visible shape.

In the case of the sportswriter, his laser is strongest which makes the chart shape protrude towards the upper left. On the other side, his middle tanden and arch are sticking out too, so the graph expands to the upper left and down to the bottom right.

Reveal your character and tendencies from the test

When you create your radar chart, you can see your character and tendencies well. Let's see some representative patterns.

The center type

First, I will explain the center type person whose center is the strongest compared to the other types of awareness. The center is the most important item among the seven body awareness types. When it's highly developed, you will have a great amount of influence. But at the same time, the center is the most difficult awareness to develop for many people.

The character of people with a strongly developed center varies depending on which other types of awareness they have. The uratenshi would be easily connected with the center. As explained earlier, the center and uratenshi complement each other. They are aligned and work around the hamstrings. This will allow you to act coherently with a steady core and mind.

Some people can be called center-laser type who have both awareness types emphasized in the radar chart. If you are this type, you must have a steady mind and see things from a wider and higher point of view. You also always tend to have goals or seek targets. You are very definite; able to point out issues accurately. Once you find a target, you are likely to go forward and reach that target sharply and coherently. If you have a developed middle tanden and arch as well in addition to a strong center, people around you will likely trust and rely on you a great deal.

The middle tanden-arch type

Next we are going to look at the middle tanden type. The middle tanden works well with the arch. These two types of awareness tend to go together.

The middle tanden is the center of passion and energy. If you have the arch as well, which allows you to have affinity for connecting with others, you will likely share your energy with others. Due to this action, the others' middle tandens will be fully charged and they can also act lively. It means your passion can be transferred to others. Therefore if a middle tanden-arch type person exists in a group, other people also tend to be passionate. Just one middle tanden-arch type can influence the whole group. People in the group will be able to exchange their emotions freely and they will trust each other passionately.

If the boss in a company is the middle tanden-arch type, his subordinates will dramatically change even within a few months. There will be no self-righteous individuals in the group. More likely there will be a friendly atmosphere. People in other groups may easily notice that and admire it, "Wow, they look so different."

The arch-laser type

Sometimes the arch works with the laser as well. When both awareness types are highly developed, that person can be called an arch-laser type.

If you are this type, you will have a strong sense of relationship. You have two different devices that can connect man-to-man and man-to-object. You can connect with other people or things strongly and accurately following a straight line. At the same time, you can also connect with them gently, warmly, and friendly following an arc. This will create the conditions for you to act intelligently, rationally, and emotionally.

The lower and middle tanden type

If you have a developed tanden both in your lower abdomen and chest, you are the lower and middle tanden type.

If you have only the lower tanden, you can be steady and won't get disturbed at critical moments. You are reliable for the people around you, which is really great. However, you might give others the impression that you are a bit unfriendly and difficult to spend time with. For example, if you got all fives for the test of the lower tanden, you must be firm and steady. But a person like this is typically no fun.

Now let's think this way. You are on a trip with a lower tanden person. You say, "There is a nice restaurant nearby. I found it in a traveler's magazine. Shall we go there?" The lower tanden person may tell you "Well, that kind of article is always an arranged tie-up with a magazine. Basically, no one can tell if the writer has enough knowledge to judge the restaurant." You must feel like "(Yeah, you are right. You are always right. But sorry, I don't want to be with you all the time.)"

However, if the middle tanden is also developed with the lower tanden, both will work in a great balance. As explained earlier, the middle tanden type tends to be easily excited about things. On a trip, this person would say "That sounds nice. Even if it's a tie-up article, at least one of 20 restaurants must be good. Not a big deal even if it's kind of disappointing. It would be rather interesting to check out a place with a high reputation." As the lower tanden is working, this type does not get excited simply or easily. However, because of the middle tanden, this person is able to enjoy life. Don't you think that a person who is reliable in a critical situation as well as always fun to be with sounds wonderful for others?

The vest-arch type

The vest is the body awareness that softens stiffness or formalities. It is ideal to combine with the center.

If you are with somebody whose center is particularly highly developed, you would feel like you always have to look up to him. That is because that person's eye level is high and you get an impression of linear stability from him. Like the person with the strong lower tanden, you might feel it's a bit hard to be with him.

If you are the center-laser type and in a group, you tend to make the atmosphere of the whole group stiff because everyone feels like you are keeping a sharp eye on them and that you see through their minds from a higher point.

However, if you have the vest as well, you can relax yourself and release unnecessary power from the shoulders. This will make others feel relaxed, too. Of course there still is a feeling or sense in others that you are looking at them sharply from a wider and higher point of view. But they would not feel something stiff or too formal.

If you are a boss with a strong vest-arch, you can support your subordinates gently and thoughtfully with empathy. In a business situation, we often complain about our bosses; "my boss never understands me." It is difficult to work and produce and perform well without a boss' support or understanding. If you have a highly developed vest and arch, you can accept your subordinate's thoughts with better understanding and support them in a better way with empathy. That will make your work or project go smoothly and successfully.

Closer look at the seven body awareness types

As you might have noticed, each section of this test has statements related to your physical aspects as well as mental aspects such as your personality or how you judge things. These are very important to evaluate your body awareness. Body awareness influences your body and simultaneously your mind as well.

Interestingly, this test shows some people are influenced by their body awareness both mentally and physically in equal balance. Others are influenced more physically but not so much mentally. On the other hand, there are people who are influenced a great deal mentally more than physically. I can say that those who are highly influenced both mentally and physically have stronger body awareness.

Athletes or other sportsmen tend to be influenced more on their body. Conversely, business professionals have more situations where their body awareness is influenced on the mental side such as judgment or human relationships. Thus it is not surprising that bigger impacts can be seen on their minds. But let me tell you this again − when your body awareness reaches the maximum level, you will be fully influenced both in your mind and body.

Now let's take a closer look at each type of body awareness.

Center

The first center-type people I think of are Ichiro and Tiger Woods. Because they are athletes, we tend to mostly see their physical aspects. However, their success would not be possible without their mental strengths.

Let's think about Ichiro's case. He crossed the ocean from Japan to the U.S. to become a Major League player. Overcoming different circumstances in a new environment, he played more games and had to travel much more than he was used to in Japan. But in only his first year, he won three titles - best batting average, most bases stolen, and the MVP award. He broke the record for the most hits in a season.

This is extraordinary. It is well beyond expectations.

In 2003, there was another famous Japanese baseball player, Hideki Matsui, who also moved to the U.S. like Ichiro did. Matsui's first year was not as successful as Ichiro's in terms of his primary role and abilities as a homerun batter. He also has physical resources that are much more than Ichiro's. But why wasn't he as successful? What was the difference between Ichiro and Matsui?

The answer is the difference between their center strengths and accuracy. Matsui's center is highly developed. But Ichiro's center is much stronger and more accurate. This strong center allows him to have a stable mental pillar in his mind and lets him focus on his way of life.

Ichiro was like this even when he was in Japan. Because of his strong personality, he has had a difficult time with media's criticism. However, even after moving to the Major League where it is a totally different environment compared to Japan, he still stayed who he was and was not distracted or overwhelmed by his surrounding circumstances. That is why he could play outstandingly from his very first year.

There are certain principals behind the results. If you know such principals, you can make changes to your body and mind, too. So, what are the principals? They are the principles underlying the seven body awareness types, including the center.

Lower Tanden

You might not have completely understood the tanden until you took the test. But now you must have a better idea of what the tanden is. You also might have a feeling that the lower tanden has opposite actions and benefits compared to those of the center.

The center gives you the body sensation of a higher center of gravity. You can feel nicely stretched out. In contrast, the lower tanden gives you the sensation of stability or fulfillment in your lower body. As written in the test, with the lower tanden, you will find physical benefits like, "I can breathe deeply and stay calm in a situation where most people would be disturbed." On the mental aspect, the lower tanden influences your personality as well. You can be a person who others can rely on in a pinch.

We normally think personality is something independent and unchangeable. This is not so. As the theory of body awareness becomes clearer, it also becomes apparent that even our personality that seems so important and unchangeable for us can be affected by the existence or non-existence of the body awareness. It means if you can obtain body awareness by practicing body awareness training, you can also change your personality with such training.

We often see mental benefits more than physical benefits in the lower tanden. But actually this awareness influences physical movements greatly as well. Especially for sumo or wrestling, the ability to control the body is directly affected by the amount of lower tanden awareness.

For example, think about two sumo wrestlers, A and B. Their body sizes are almost the same. But A looks to have a more stable and weighty lower body. You might instantly feel A must be stronger than B. It is usually true. Conversely, if there is a sumo wrestler with a thin lower body, high center of gravity, and his body seems to be stretched vertically, which means he is the center type, he would not be stable enough as a sumo wrestler. His match tends to be nervous and on edge. That's because sumo is a typical lower tanden type sport.

How about judo? It is a sport that requires wrestling. However, not only foreign wrestlers but also Japanese wrestlers tend to stand straight without lowering their hips like sumo wrestlers do. Judo is a center type sport. Of course there may be some judo wrestlers who are like sumo wrestlers with lower hips and weighty legs. But if you watch international competitions such as the Olympics, you will find many sharp-framed center type wrestlers, especially in Europe.

In the earliest days of the internationalization of judo, there was a Dutch wrestler who stood out in the history of Japanese judo. Anton Geesink; he won the gold medal, defeating the strongest Japanese wrestler at the Tokyo Olympics in Japan - judo's home country. Geesink played a large part in the internationalization of judo. He was a typical center type.

Yasuhiro Yamashita, one of the most successful judo competitors, was a wrestler who had both the center and the lower tanden. To put it the other way around, he was very strong—he won 203 consecutive victories—because he had both the center and the lower tanden. The strength born from the center not to lose the core line and the strength born from the lower tanden to place him firmly into the earth - Yamashita had these two strengths.

Middle Tanden

If you have tried the test, you must understand that the middle tanden is the center of 'energy and passion.' This is the primary feature. Its mental benefit is to provide you with motivation. As written in the test, if you have the middle tanden, you will become more active and be passionate when you love somebody. The influences of the middle tanden can be seen not only in personality but also in various matters such as work, as well as art, music, or cooking.

The middle tanden lets you instantly feel something beautiful before you think of it in your head. When you eat something delicious, the middle tanden lets you say, "It's good!" without thinking. On the other hand, if you are lacking the middle tanden, you would not be able to say, "It's good," until someone asks you if it's good or not. A person who has the middle tanden shows a big smile and expresses how good that food or cooking is before analyzing it technically. If there is a person like this around you, you and the other people would feel good, too. If you were a host of a party and found this type of person there, you'd be glad that you had invited that person to your party.

In contrast, being gloomy is a symptom of the deficiency of the middle tanden. Someone who is socially withdrawn has no middle tanden or only a little of it. We often say, "Chest up, stand up straight," to those who look downcast and have no energy. That is because we know the middle tanden intuitively.

The actions of the middle tanden can be seen as your body shape, movements, or even as body expressions. In fact, if you see photos of popular politicians or entertainers, they look full of confidence that comes from their chests. In other words, if they didn't look that way, they couldn't attract people at all. John F. Kennedy was a politician who had a highly developed middle tanden. With his strong middle tanden, people were attracted by him and had expectations like, "Yes, he can do something."

In the field of baseball, the legendary homerun king in the US, Babe Ruth, was a person who had a super middle tanden. When looking at managers, Tony La Russa had a great middle tanden, too. He became only the second manager ever to win the World Series for both National and American league teams. Ruth and La Russa; they both had a strong arch as well which allowed them to have tight relationships with their fans and teammates. They were passionate and strongly motivated. These factors helped Ruth's remarkable batting performance and La Russa's excellent management in combining all powers of his teammates and defeating other teams.

Special Column: Where is your inner strength?

There may be few women who tap their chest while saying "Rely on me!" However, a gutsy mom has exactly that kind of image. Guts have the meaning of courage or fortitude. The physical meaning is entrails located below the diaphragm where it is very close to the locations of the middle and lower tanden. Especially, the lower tanden is within the guts. In this sense, the gutsy mom can be described as a woman who has both the middle and lower tanden. Having fortitude or being steady is a benefit of the lower tanden. Having courage or being positive or aggressive is an action from the middle tanden.

Arch

Arch is a body awareness you can instantly recognize in action. The arch allows you to connect with people in a warm gentle relationship. By contrast, the relationship connected by the laser is sharp and tense. Among the seven body awareness types, the arch is the one you can see the training effects of most easily.

The effects of the arch are as written in the test. First, you enjoy speaking in front of people. When speaking to a large number of people, we usually become nervous and even feel like running away. Speaking coaches suggest you think that they are just pumpkins. This may reduce your nervousness, but it is not really fun to speak to pumpkins. However, if you draw an imaginary arc from yourself to the audience before you appear in front of them as if you are connected to them, your nervousness will decrease but your affinity will increase naturally. You will have more fun speaking to the audience.

If the arch has been developed and you realize that you have it, you will have confidence about getting along with people. But if you have a problem with human relationships at work, or if you cannot be open to your boss or a colleague who tries to direct you, you may be lacking the arch.

Vest

Let's make sure where the lines of the vest go. In each side of your shoulders, the vest goes on the muscle called trapezius. This muscle can also be called the 'stiff shoulder muscle'. It is located on the bottom of the back of your head, the back of your neck, on your shoulders and your back. It consists of the large muscles that together are shaped like a diamond, located on your upper back.

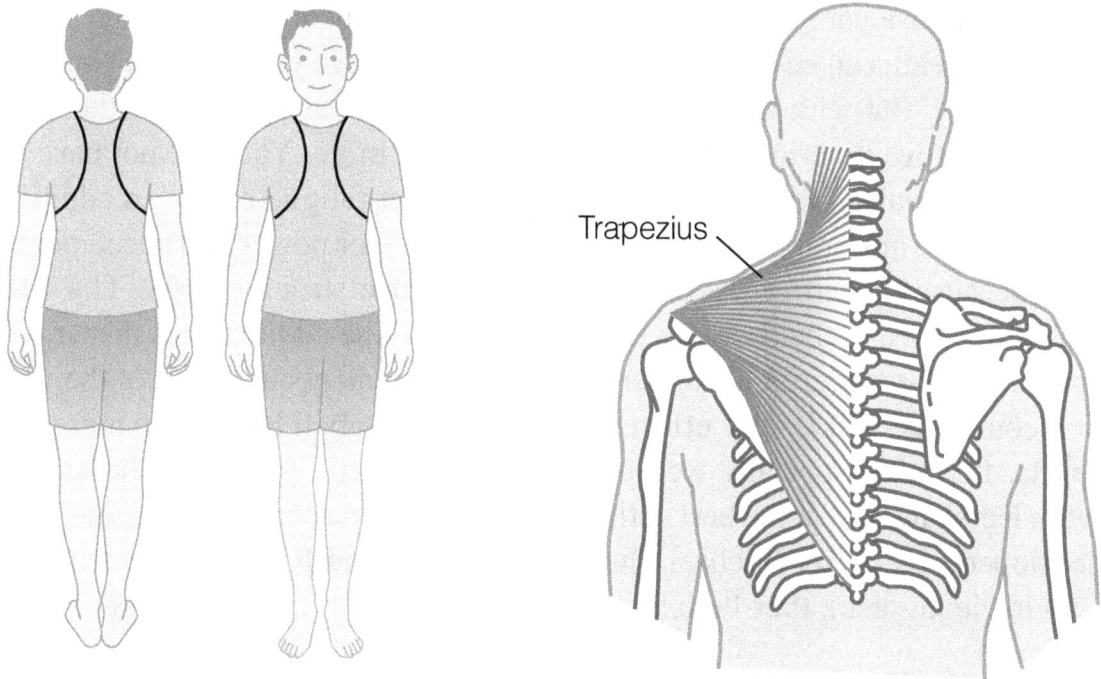

Trapezius

The vest activates these trapezius muscles. An activated muscle means you can repeatedly contract or relax it more sensitively. In other words, the muscle is standing by to immediately contract or relax as needed. This is standby tension that has the status of no stiffness. Thus if the vest is appropriately developed, you will be relieved from the stiffness in your shoulder, neck, and back.

If the vest is further developed, the rib cage becomes more flexible. In this stage, your upper body can be moved naturally and softly. As a result, extra effort in your shoulders will of course be gone and you will have no tension in your shoulders, upper arms, and elbows. This will allow you to breathe deeply with no effort. Here, 'tension in your shoulders, upper arms, and elbows' refers to the body, but this actually is related to the mental side as well. When you put a lot of effort on your trapezius and your rib cage is stiff, you will feel inflexible. People around you feel the same about you. This will likely make your relationships with others inflexible, too.

Let me explain this more. You create an inflexible impression by yourself. Others see and catch your inflexibility. They became tense and inflexible, too. An inflexible relationship is created in this situation. However, the vest can avoid creating this undesirable cycle.

If you can use your trapezius smoothly and freely using the vest, the shoulder blades underneath can be flexible as well. You might move your arms at your shoulder joints only. But with the vest, you can control your arms from further inside. This will improve functions of your arms more and more. You will not have stiffness in your shoulder which means you will not feel fatigue easily. In addition to this, the flexible movements of the rib cage make further power and speed possible. This is because the rib cage's flexibility can produce strong energy. The energy will be transferred to the shoulder blades and arms. The addition and dispersion of Ichiro's muscular power in his upper body is the advantageous effect of the vest.

Of course the vest is very effective not only in baseball but also in many kinds of sports. It works especially well in ball sports, swimming, and fighting sports. Clayton Kershaw, one of the best active Major League baseball pitchers, has a highly developed vest. Also, Michael Phelps (Swimmer) and Rickson Gracie (Martial artist, Gracie jiu-jitsu); they both have incredible vests.

Special Column: The Secret of the Cheetah's Speed

The cheetah is the fastest land animal known. Probably most readers have seen this animal's amazing run on TV or a video. The ones we've seen often show the cheetah's speed not only at actual speed but also in slow motion. When we see it in slow motion, we are very impressed with the performance and notice that the cheetah's scapula (shoulder blades) and rib cage look like they are rotating.

The fact is, from the viewpoint of biomechanics, there are two different shifting rotational motions at its rib cage and scapula. The rib cage rotates while each rib bone moves and shifts individually. This is called the rib's shifting rotational motion. The scapula rotates in a slower cycle but it is coordinated with the shifting cycle of the rib cage. At top speed, the scapula and rib cage rotate in almost the same cycle. They are perfectly balanced with each other. These two shifting rotational motions produce muscular energy. This energy is amplified and transferred to the ground via the front limbs. That is their motion structure. (The back limbs are not relevant here.)

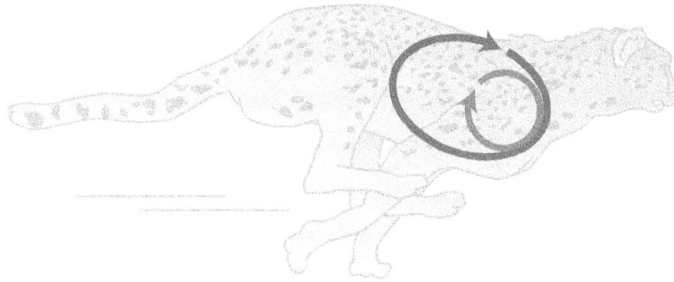

When we look at these amazing motions, we have a tremendous feeling about them. In order to make such a movement, it is necessary to have body awareness just like the ones in the human body. In this case, the vest is the one we need to be aware of.

For a human, the vest works to improve the throwing or pitching motions of baseball as well as the stroking motion of swimming. But let's think back to ancient times when we were four-limbed animals, like a cheetah. We should have experienced the vest as a profound device to create outstanding performance in our forelimbs. When we realize this, we notice the great possibility hidden in our bodies. We can even have a similar feeling about the cheetah's amazing performance. Furthermore, we will have a strong desire to think about ourselves as having greater potential. Don't you think so?

Uratenshi (Back Push)

Uratenshi (Back Push) is the body awareness that influences your body and movements more than your mind. As written in the test, the uratenshi allows you to make a great standing posture with the high center of gravity that many people long for.

For example, look at the walking of top models or Hollywood actresses. You will notice how attractively and gracefully they walk. The uratenshi is the awareness that produces such a nice walking style.

The development of the uratenshi increases the power output of the hamstrings and the gluteus maximus (the muscles in the buttocks). This allows you to press the ground down strongly and long enough with your heels while the backside of your knee is properly stretched. With this style, you have a high center of gravity. You can shift your weight smoothly. When swinging your leg forward, your knee is nicely stretched to press down on the ground with your heel. That is why you can make a smooth and graceful stride while maintaining a high center of gravity.

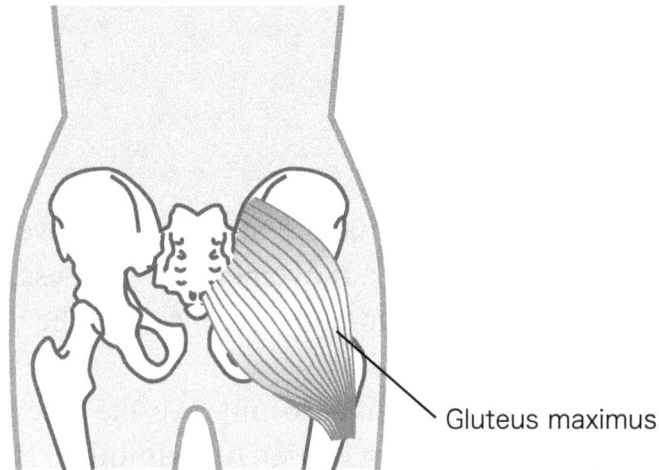

Gluteus maximus

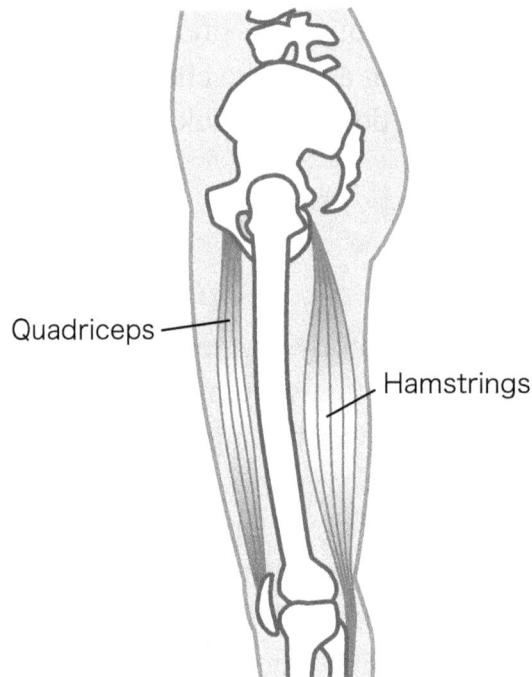

Quadriceps

Hamstrings

On the other hand, if your uratenshi is not active, you instead use your front thighs to walk. It makes your walk look ugly even if you are wearing nice fancy high heels. When kicking the ground with your back leg, your knee is not stretching out enough. It is bent and your heel rises too soon. This doesn't look beautiful at all.

A firm, smooth, graceful walk with the high center of gravity, in which the center works, requires that you firmly hit the ground with your heels with the knee not bending. You touch the ground from the heel. Walking with bent knees and a lower center of gravity is totally opposite to the graceful walk of top models. However, if you develop the uratenshi, you will definitely be able to walk like them.

As described in the previous chapter, the lines of the uratenshi go along your hamstrings. Regardless of the length or size of your legs, a nice body requires nice fit hamstrings. Look at top marathon runners. For example, Naoko Takahashi (a former runner in Japan) and Paula Radcliffe (England); their bodies are thin and perfectly in shape and their hamstrings are excellently developed.

Among ordinary people, some become or stay skinny using just a diet. It cannot be said they have a well-shaped body. A real well-shaped body means a body with the highly developed uratenshi that can develop your hamstrings where you support your weight using the back thighs to walk. This is like the body of a top runner of track and field.

The mental benefit of the uratenshi is that it provides you with motivation to go forward. The elements that work as a brake will decrease both in your body and mind.

Laser

You will understand the features of the laser and the arch very well by comparing them to each other. The arch has an action of love and affinity which allows you to be friendly. On the other hand, the laser connects you to people or an object geometrically, accurately and strictly. Therefore, if the laser is highly developed, you can aim at something more accurately and sharper. Just like a laser gunsight, in order to aim at something it is best to make a straight line to it. The feature of the laser as a body awareness technique is exactly the same as a laser is to physical matters.

Compared to the arch that creates affinity, the laser produces the impression of rationality as well as a dry or cool image. As written in the test "my gaze is strong and sharp, " you can think that your eye gaze is made based on the laser that you make.

Another statement "I can find a target (thing or person) in a crowd quickly," is the best way to find out if you have the laser or not because the answer varies most depending on people. In my case, I am good at finding a person in a crowd. I am quite tall, so people can easily find me. But when I meet someone somewhere, I usually find them first.

The third statement was about your behavior. It shows an effect of the laser appearing on your mental side. If you have the developed laser, you would feel like "I must do this," as if you are connected to your goal with an invisible string. You will likely overcome difficulties and can reach your goal. Furthermore, because you are always looking at the goal, you can quickly point out obstacles or problems as well.

The laser allows you to have a strong gaze with the feeling that the target should be tightly connected to you, and you can point your laser toward various directions. For example, when you walk in a crowd, you can see a line in between people which allows you to go through without bumping into others. Another example is; when you are in a line for a cashier, you can easily find the best line that flows most smoothly.

Chapter 4

Master Body Awareness
The Takaoka Training Methods

How to awaken the power of the human body

The most important key is to loosen your body

In this chapter, I introduce you to some actual training methods, the YURU EXERCISES, to develop your body awareness. You may feel like "OK, now I know which awareness I want to improve. I am ready to learn how." Unfortunately, starting the practices without enough knowledge will result in gaining only a few benefits. In order to create the structure of your body awareness and get the full benefits from it, you must build up the fundamental parts first. YURU EXERCISES allow you to prepare such basic parts while practicing to develop your body awareness.

Assume that you will be creating the center in your body. If you maintain an image of the center and practice the exercises in this book, you will eventually have the centerline in your subconscious. To understand this, you can think about how you learn a foreign language. You repeat a word or phrase over and over again until you memorize it. That will eventually stay in your brain. Just like this, if you keep thinking of a strong image of something repeatedly, it will stay in your subconscious even when you are not thinking about it consciously.

Body awareness works exactly in the same way. It is developed by repetition. For example, to create the center that is the vertical straight-line awareness, you first need to have an image of such a line. If you practice taking that line into your body, gradually something similar will be created. Of course it is not so easy to do. But if you imagine the centerline over and over again and put it into your mind and body, that line will surely be developed in your body.

However, there is one problem here. The center you will have created from following the above will be very rigid. You cannot realize all the benefits that I have discussed in this book. One of the benefits from the center is that you will be able to see things from a wider and higher point of view. At the same time, you will notice details but you won't care about too many small things. But if you imagine the centerline by only thinking about its shape, that line will be inflexible. Possibly this will cause you to care about every little thing and you will point them out arrogantly and speak as if you are looking down on others. The authentic center should make you notice the details, but at the same time, you can recognize what's more important and what's less important. This will allow you to forget about or forgive small things. That is the tremendous benefit of the authentic center.

Conversely, if you can see the small things well but you only talk them down to others, you will likely be an annoying person. Is there anyone who is like this around you? Very arrogant, too much detail, and speaks as if you are an inferior. You might become like this if you try to take the center into your body without enough preparation.

What is the difference between a fake center and the authentic center?

The answer is whether you are loosened up or not. In other words, the body awareness is affected whether or not your body and mind are deeply relaxed. If neither is deeply relaxed but you created the center-like awareness in your subconscious, then you will become a person who cares about every little thing and talks down to others. Again, the point is to loosen up your body and mind first. If you immediately begin with simple image training without loosening yourself, only rigid results (awareness) can be seen which reflect your body and mind. In order to create the authentic body awareness, the most important preparation will be completely loosening your body and mind, and becoming deeply relaxed.

In the first half of this chapter, I introduce you to the most basic types of YURU EXERCISES to loosen up your body. These are the common methods for developing all body awareness types. Start with these exercises, and then go onto other types of YURU EXERCISES to strengthen each type of body awareness, as will be explained in the second half of this chapter. Following this order (i.e. establish a fundamental state where your body and mind are both nice and loose first, then go onto each specific exercise next), each awareness can be created in an ideal form and condition. Another important note is, when you first try to practice the specific exercise for each body awareness type, please be sure to try the one for developing the center first, then try the one for the lower tanden. This is the most ideal order to create an overall excellent body awareness.

YURU EXERCISES - Powerful Relaxation Techniques - More effective than simply stretching!

There are many relaxation methods to relax your body and mind. The methods I introduce here are called YURU EXERCISES. YURU consists of YURU THEORY, a thought process that is conceived based on the study of philosophy and science. It also consists of YURU PRACTICE, a comprehensive body and mind training system that was established to realize YURU THEORY. YURU EXERCISES are positioned under YURU PRACTICE as the most representative and basic introductory method for the public to this entire system. By practicing YURU everyday, we can train, improve, and grow the true nature of ourselves in all aspects of intelligence, emotions, and physical and mental ability throughout our entire life – that is called the YURU WAY.

The YURU EXERCISES introduced in this book are for loosening up your body and mind and developing your body awareness, but are also helpful as supplementary treatments to cure diseases or for conditioning your body and mind to prevent diseases. I would like to talk about how the YURU EXERCISES would work to get these benefits in other places, but let's focus on the basic topic now for you to get to know more of the main subject of this book, 'body awareness' and how the YURU EXERCISES are beneficial to develop your body awareness.

YURU EXERCISES are configured for each body part. With a variety of methods such as using onomatopoeic words, rubbing the targeted body parts, stimulating acupuncture points, and breathing methods, the YURU EXERCISES remove body stiffness and cure brain fatigue very smoothly and bring you back to a state where you can experience the true nature of yourself–a comfortably loosened body and mind. It is an innovative unique exercise method you've never experienced before.

Most of the YURU EXERCISES are named using Japanese onomatopoeia; "pura-pura," "mozo-mozo," and so on. When you practice the YURU EXERCISES, using onomatopoeic words is very useful. It makes your movements improve significantly and helps your body become more relaxed. This is because when you use the onomatopoeia, the motor, sensory, language, and pre-frontal areas, cerebellum, and basal ganglia, of your brain are all linked and working together. This will allow you to loosen every muscle of your body, even very difficult parts such as your blood vessels, rib cage, and internal organs. It definitely helps your health and toned body. You might have seen Japanese onomatopoeic words in Manga. But for those who are not familiar with them, English translations and illustrations are included in this book. Japanese onomatopoeic words have a variety of kinds and are truly fun words to learn. Laughing and smiling are two great keys to success. For even more fun, try and use the Japanese onomatopoeia while loosening your body.

In the first half of this chapter, the basic types of YURU EXERCISES —the common methods for developing all body awareness types— are introduced. By practicing these exercises, you can expect to obtain a better body and mind condition and your brain and body fatigue will be smoothly eased. As a result, you can get ready to have more benefits from other types of YURU EXERCISE which are designed for each body awareness type specifically.

YURU EXERCISES are easy to start for anybody. Try each exercise for about 30 seconds to 2 minutes as a good start. With appropriate and accustomed practice, your body and mind condition will improve. You can be healthier and relaxed in your daily life. Your stress will be eased. You can naturally maintain your health and energy all by yourself with your own tremendous power.

BASIC YURU EXERCISES - common to all body awareness types -

Let's get started with the basic YURU EXERCISES which are beneficial to all of body awareness types. YURU EXERCISES can be categorized into four groups, FLOOR YURU - practice while lying down, SITTING YURU - practice while seated, STANDING YURU - practice while standing, and BREATHING YURU - practice while focusing on your breathing. We will start with the easiest and most beneficial one, the FLOOR YURU!

HIP Mozo-Mozo EXERCISE

Gently loosen the hip area while lying down. Ease fatigue in the hip area. Prevent the lower back ache.

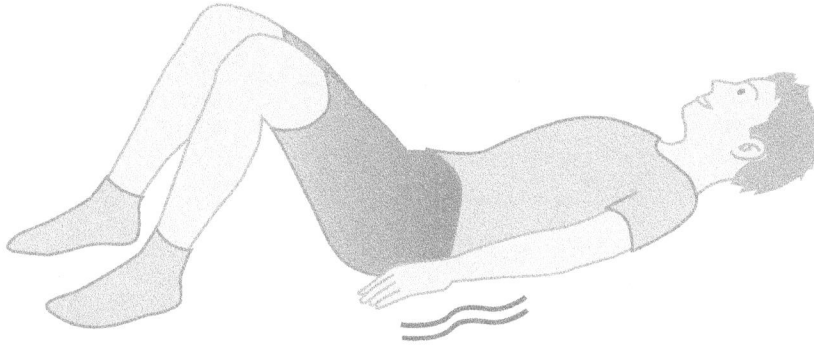

1) Lay on your back. Completely relax.
2) Pull your knees up. Your hands are by your side. Allow your legs to naturally spread apart. Release all your tension.
3) While saying, "mozo-mozo," slowly and gently move your hips right and left to loosen them up. Keep your buttocks (lumber spine) slightly and softly touching the floor.

Note: Make sure to release all the tension in your entire body, especially around your hips. When moving your hips, there is no space between your buttocks (lumber spine) and the floor. Just relax as if you are gently rubbing them on the floor.

Japanese Onomatopoeia

mozo-mozo	Describes something wriggling, wiggling or twisting.	

YURU EXERCISE - Basic - FLOOR YURU

Kozo Calf

CALF Kozo-Kozo EXERCISE

Easy calves massage while lying down. Better blood circulation. Ease fatigue and swelling in the legs. Warm up the whole lower body.

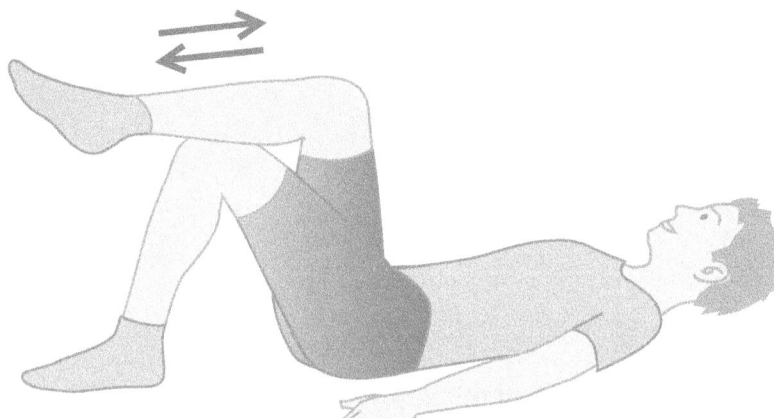

1) Lay on your back. Pull your knees up.
2) Put your right calf on your left knee. Relax.
3) While saying, "kozo-kozo," move your right calf back and forth and find the right spot (an area where you might feel a little pain but comfortable enough). Keep massaging until your calf is loosened.
4) Switch your legs and repeat.

Note: Do not press your calf too hard. Release the tension in your leg as much as possible. Only feel gravity on your leg. No extra force is needed. The most important thing is to feel comfortable and allow yourself to enjoy the sensation.

Japanese Onomatopoeia

Kozo-kozo	"Kozo-kozo" sounds very much like a typical Japanese onomatopoeia, but actually it's an invented word by the author. Japanese people say "hiza kozou (knee boy)" for the top of the knee because it looks like a boy's head. The Takaoka's unique word "kozo-kozo" came from "kozou."

ANKLE CROSSING EXERCISE

Crossing ankles to loosen them up. Ease fatigue in the ankles through the lower body.

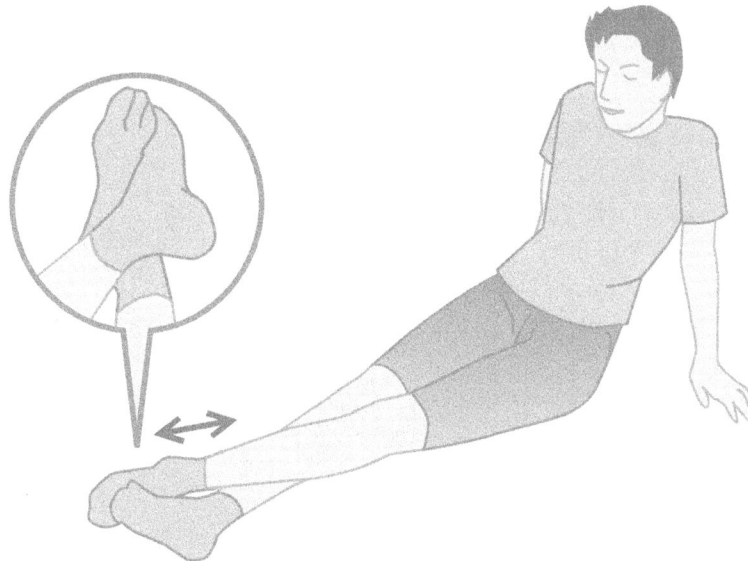

This exercise can be done on the sofa, but sitting on the hard floor is more appropriate and recommended. If your work requires walking or standing all day or for long hours, you can get rid of the fatigue in your ankles and throughout your lower body.

1) Sit on the floor. Straighten your legs naturally. Put your hands behind you. Straighten your elbows naturally. Release all the tension in your shoulder and neck. Completely relax your entire body.
2) Put your left foot on your right foot. Cross your ankles and relax. Your upper (left) baby toe is invisible under the lower (right) baby toe.
3) No tension is needed. While saying, "Feels good. Feels good." gently pull up your left leg and release it. Pull up and release to massage your ankles.
4) Switch your legs and repeat.

Note: You should not feel any pain in the crossing part. Move your legs gently. Wearing soft socks helps avoiding discomfort.

YURU EXERCISE   - Basic - SITTING YURU

Mozo Neck

LEAN BACK NECK Mozo-Mozo EXERCISE

Stimulate the acupuncture point between the back neck and head using a chair back-rest. Ease the brain fatigue. Activate your brain more. Recommended for business people who are working on a chair all day and have fewer chances to do exercises.

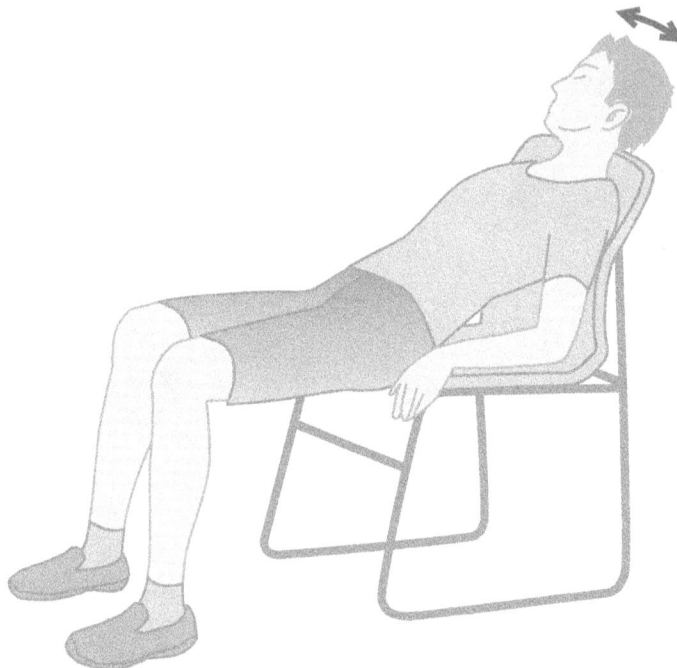

1) Sit down on a chair that has a backrest. Lean back and move your hips forward until the hollow of your upper neck (the hollow at the border of your neck and head) goes right on the top of the backrest. Find the right point by adjusting your hips back and forth.
2) Place your back head and neck to rest naturally on the backrest. Completely relax. While saying, "mozo-mozo," move your neck right and left, right and left.

Note: Too much motion can cause a neck injury. Gently move your neck only about half or one inch (about 1 or 2.5cm). You should feel comfortable but not a pain.

Japanese Onomatopoeia

mozo-mozo	Describes something wriggling, wiggling or twisting.	

SIT BONE Mozo-Mozo SITTING EXERCISE

Loosen the pelvic floor muscle and the erector spinae muscles while sitting on a chair. Activate the iliopsoas and inner muscles around the spine. Recommended for business people who are sitting in a chair all day and have fewer chances to do exercises.

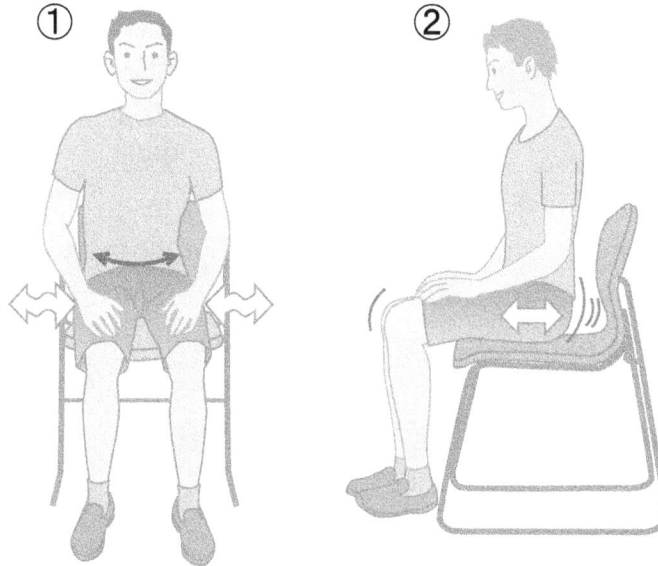

1) Sit on a chair. While saying, "mozo-mozo," move your hips right and left, right and left, until you find your sitting bones located in each center of your buttocks.
2) Once you found your sitting bones, move them as if you are rubbing them on the chair, first one side then the other side. Keep rubbing.
3) Next, gently move your sitting bones back and forth. Move very smoothly on two imaginary short rails attached on the chair.
4) Again, move your sitting bones and rub them on the chair, first one side then the other side. Keep rubbing. When you do this, imagine that you are building vertebral bones (spine) one by one from the bottom to the top.

Note: Release all the tension in your torso. Completely relax. Allow your torso to move naturally like waving according to the movement of your buttocks.

Japanese Onomatopoeia

mozo-mozo	Describes something wriggling, wiggling or twisting.	

WRIST Pura-Pura EXERCISE

From here, I will teach you the STANDING YURU. Let's get started with the most basic type – the WRIST Pura-Pura EXERCISE. "Pura-pura" means swinging or swaying.

First, gently rub one hand and wrist with the other hand. Repeat with the opposite hand. The tip here is to say, "Feels good. Feels good." You might think "What? That's embarrassing. There shouldn't be any difference whether I say this or not." If you think something like this, instead say quietly "Feels bad... Feels bad..." You will have an unpleasant feeling coming from your hands even before repeating it five times or so. Words have such power. If you say "Feels good. Feels good." your body will likely be in a good condition. There is a close relationship between our mind and body. When you are feeling good, your body reacts in a good way such as the metabolism or blood flow in capillary vessels increasing.

After you rub your hands and wrists well, shake them to feel even better. As you have rubbed those parts, those areas must be sensitive. You will notice that your wrists and hands are really dangling loosely.

How is it?

I think you'll feel like those parts are released, loosened, and relaxed. In fact, 'release, loosen, and relax' are the main purposes of this exercise. The WRIST Pura-Pura EXERCISE is designed for loosening the wrists and hands only. But in our body, the center goes through up and down, the middle tanden in the chest, the lower tanden in the lower abdomen, and so on. It means we should loosen our whole body, not just our wrists or hands.

In general, when thinking about loosening the body, many people think stretching is the way to do it. However, although stretching allows you to expand the range of motion in your joints and stretch muscles, it's not so much about releasing or loosening your entire body.

For example, stretching the shoulders or the legs is an exercise for those parts of the body such as the shoulder blades or hip joints that contain large muscles. A muscle that is stretched and then released will be slightly longer. As a result, the stretched muscle will be loosened slightly. That is how stretching works. When focusing on loosening the body, it works a little bit, but doesn't affect the smaller or inner muscles so much throughout the body.

On the other hand, YURU EXERCISES are shaking motions. They also include wiggling and twisting motions. So, more precisely, I can say these exercises are shaking and loosening motions. These motions work for the small muscles deep inside your body. They allow you to loosen every single part. When focusing on loosening the entire body, more benefits can be expected from these motions rather than just from stretching.

YURU EXERCISE - Basic - STANDING YURU

WRIST Pura-Pura EXERCISE

Loosen the wrists, hands, and shoulder areas. Ease the fatigue throughout your hands and the entire length of your arms. Gain more functional and activated hands and arms.

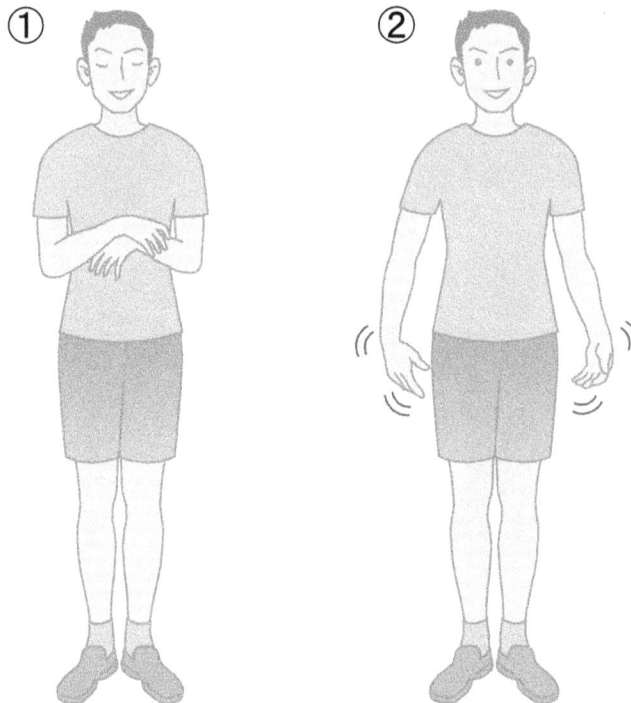

1) Stand with your legs relaxed and apart. Rub one hand and wrist with the other hand, saying, "Feels good. Feels good"—repeat with the opposite hand.
2) Shake your wrists as if your entire hands are loosely dangling. Feel that your wrists are totally loosened and relaxed while saying "pura-pura, pura-pura."

Japanese Onomatopoeia

pura-pura	Describes something swinging or swaying, etc.	

To make your body more controllable

After you are done with the YURU EXERCISE for the wrists, how do your wrists feel?

Some people may say their wrists are warm now. Other may feel the blood vessels are open, the blood flows from the wrists to the hands, and feel like their hands are swollen. If you have this kind of sensation, it means you had a lot of tension and fatigue in your wrists and hands.

The YURU EXERCISES start with the wrists and move to the forearms, elbows, upper arms, shoulders, and eventually go to the top of the head and the tip of the toes. First, make sure to rub gently the body part to be loosened just like you did on your wrists. The targeted body part will start loosening up and simultaneously you can have a higher and more sensitive body sensation around that part.

Now, let's do it for another part.

Rub your left shoulder with your right hand. Say, "Feels good. Feels good." Gently rub the areas around the shoulder joints and trapezius muscles while lowering your left shoulder slightly. When your shoulder becomes nice and comfortable, lift the shoulder up and release. Again, up and release. Don't use too much effort. Keep your shoulder up and release as it becomes very loose and relaxed. After you repeat this several times, compare your body sensation in your left shoulder and right shoulder.

How is it?

Don't you think your left shoulder is more deeply sensitive? This is very important. To loosen and appropriately condition your body, it is necessary to deepen your body sensations first.

It may sound too technical, but let me explain. In each part of our body, there are nerves that are connected to the sensory area in your brain. There is also a motor area controlled by the nervous system called the efferent nerve. The sensory and motor areas are closely linked. In this sequence, increasing the body sensation deeply means increasing the ability to control that body part. Through the WRIST Pura-Pura EXERCISE or the above experiments on your shoulder, you might have already realized that your body sensation has deeply increased by rubbing that part. Just rub a body part while saying, "Feels good. Feels good." This allows you to control your body better.

Great athletes also loosen their bodies

The main motion of YURU EXRCISES is not just rubbing. It is rather shaking to loosen your body. You might be skeptical about this and think, "Just shaking and loosening? Does it really work?" I can confidently say that nothing works better than YURU EXRCISES to deeply loosen your body and make your body and mind healthy and relaxed.

Now, let's think this way. Have you ever seen the shaking motion to loosen a body anywhere?

Yes, that is top level swimmers! Most of them are loosening up their bodies before starting the races. They are very good examples you can easily understand. Also, there is another athlete who loosens up his body. This may be a difficult question even if you're a big sports fan. Do you know who he is?

The answer is Michael Jordan. No one would notice but he used to keep loosening inside his body even in the middle of games. This gave rise to the highest body and mind condition and showed us a variety of super performances such as his Air Walk or his incredible come-from-behind win shots. His unique motion is a perfect example of the shaking and loosening motion.

The swimmer, Michael Phelps, also shakes his body before the start of a race. The golfer, Tiger Woods, wiggles his hands, arms, and body before his shots, too. He uses this motion to loosen and reset his entire body. Once he fully realizes the loosened sensation, he then goes into the swing motion. Just like them, many top athletes unconsciously use the shaking and loosening motions to bring out their best performance. The best athletes in history had this same tendency. They were shaking, swinging and swaying every spare moment they had.

For another example, the legendary sprinter, Carl Lewis - he is one of them. When looking at his photo, he may not seem very relaxed. However, he used to spend a long time before each race doing shaking and loosening motions and stretching at a sub field.

Among Japanese athletes, the judo wrestler Yasuhiro Yamashita, who won nine consecutive All-Japan Judo Championships, was shaking and loosening his body all the time. His continuous swaying motion might seem uncomfortable and restless for others, but he was an impressive athlete who won 203 consecutive matches. Even though he looked like he was swaying all the time, I think nobody thought he was a restless person.

A giant in the field of karate, Masutatsu Oyama, who founded Kyokushin Karate, shook his body even more than Yamashita. Every muscle of his body was very soft. But, when needed, they contracted immediately and strongly. Because of this big gap - softness and hardness - incredible power can be produced.

I can also see that the super sprinter, Usain Bolt, who amazingly achieved world records in the short-distance races, was always moving and shaking his body to completely loosen it up even at the competition sites.

As mentioned above, if you look at the fields of sports or martial arts, you will notice that people who always use the shaking and loosening motions to loosen their bodies and minds tend to be able to produce great athletic performances. They are also tough and clever. YURU EXERCISES are innovative training methods that were designed based on scientific studies of the mechanisms employed in shaking and loosening motions. These exercises can provide anybody the highest benefits.

Now, I introduce you to more of the STANDING YURU. These are also very easy and beneficial. Enjoy your practice!

YURU EXERCISE - Basic - STANDING YURU

Neba Feet

FEET Neba-Neba WALKING EXERCISE

Loosen the whole body while walking.

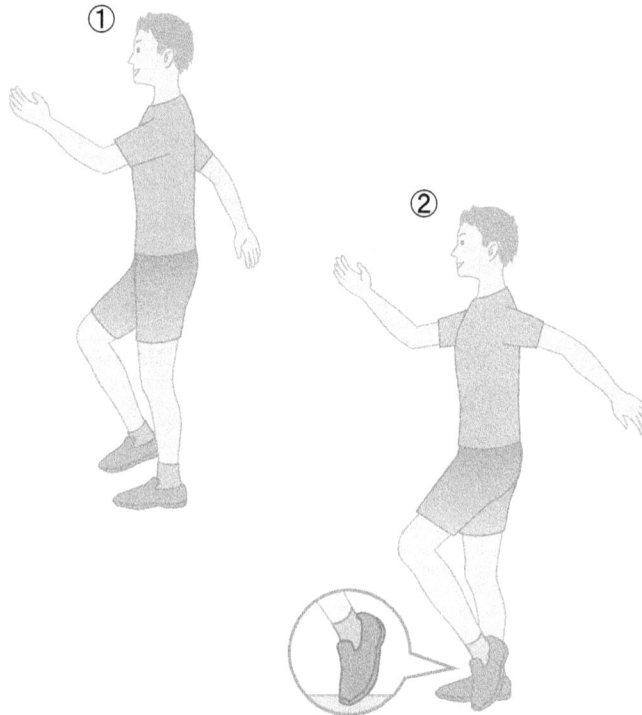

1) Walk in place (without moving forward), on a spot while swinging your arms naturally. Imagine that your whole body is totally loosened.
2) Keep walking in place on the spot, but raise up your heels only. Walk as if your feet are sticky and your toes are completely stuck to the floor, saying, "neba-neba, neba-neba." Once you get used to this, swing your arms broadly and keep walking on the spot.

Note: Imagine that your abs, hips, and back are totally loosened.

Japanese Onomatopoeia

neba-neba	Describes something sticky, tacky or gooey that clings easily.	

STIFF SHOULDER Gyuu Dosah EXERCISE

Loosen the shoulder area. Release the stress. Create the center.

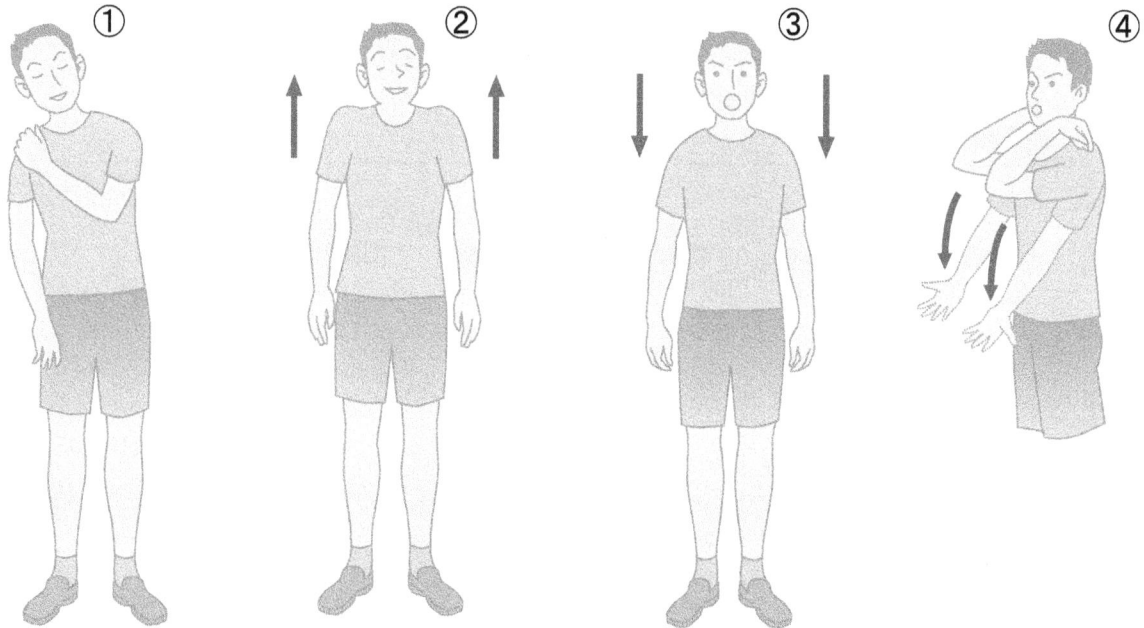

1) Slightly lower your left shoulder. Gently rub the left side of your trapezius muscle while saying, "Feels good. Feels good." Slightly lower your right shoulder. Gently rub the right side of your trapezius muscle while saying, "Feels good. Feels good."
2) Pull up and squeeze your shoulders while saying "gyuu."
3) Release your shoulders as if you let something heavy drop down while saying "dosah." Repeat "gyuu" and "dosah" several times until you feel comfortable with your shoulders.
4) As you inhale, fold your arms upwards. As you exhale, straighten them down while saying "duwah." Imagine you have a heavy burden on your shoulders and you put it down vigorously. Repeat all three movements, saying "gyuu," "dosah" and "duwah" several times.

Note: When you say "duwah," think of your internal organs dropping down inside your body.

Japanese Onomatopoeia

gyuu	Describes squeezing, being squeezed or being wrung.	
dosah	Describes a large number of objects or a heavy object being dumped, put down or dropped into place.	
duwah	Describes a rather large number of objects or a large amount of liquid flowing, splashing or vigorously falling down.	

SHOULDER Yuttari ROLLING EXERCISE

Roll to loosen the shoulders. Release stiffness and fatigue in the shoulder area. Increase the function of the shoulders, the shoulder blades, and the rib cage.

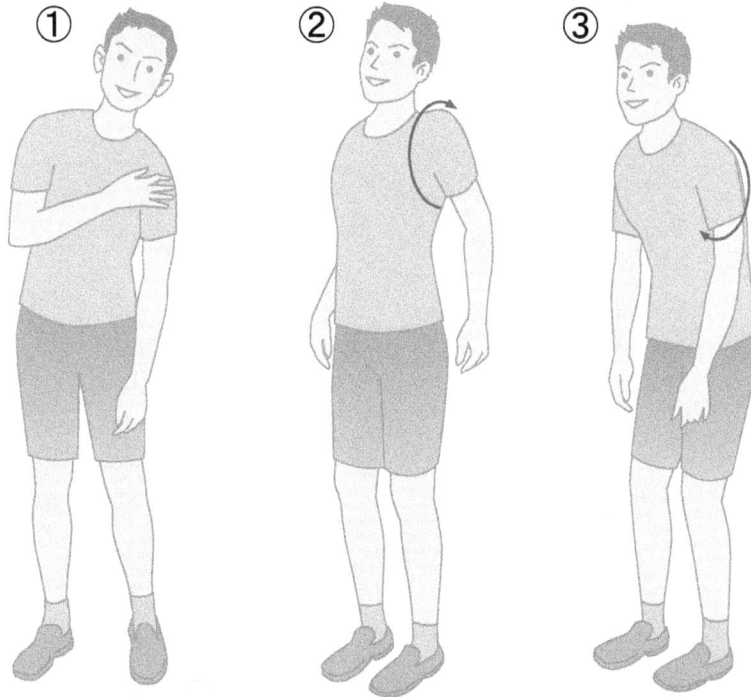

1) Slightly lower your left shoulder. Gently rub your left shoulder area while saying, "Feels good. Feels good." Slightly lower your right shoulder. Gently rub your right shoulder area while saying, "Feels good. Feels good."
2) Roll your shoulders slowly, gently and widely from front to upward and then to back, saying "yuttari, yuttari" as you roll your shoulders.

Note: Imagine your shoulders are totally loosened up and relaxed. When you roll your shoulders, move your upper body as if you are stretching yourself.

Japanese Onomatopoeia

yuttari	Describes behaving calmly with plenty of leeway or moving slowly, loosely, spaciously.	

YURU EXERCISE - Basic - STANDING YURU

Mozo Shoulder Blade

SHOULDER BLADE Mozo-Mozo EXERCISE

Loosen the shoulders area focusing on shoulder blades

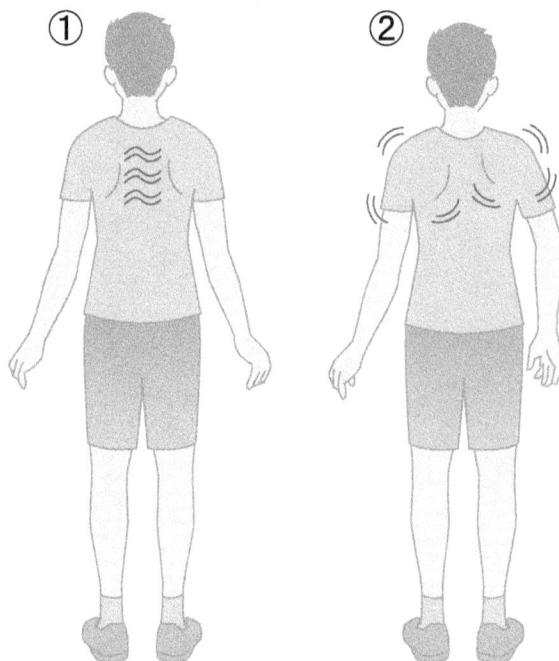

1) Wriggle your shoulder blades to loosen them, while saying, "mozo-mozo."
2) Wriggle your shoulder blades and the area between them. Loosen all the muscles and tendons around your shoulder blades.
3) Move your arms and shoulder blades as if your shoulder blades are a sliding door that opens and closes very smoothly and gently, while saying "susuu."

Note: Imagine the entire area around your shoulder blades is totally loosened.

Japanese Onomatopoeia

mozo-mozo	Describes something wriggling, wiggling or twisting.	
susuu	Describes something moving silently and smoothly with almost no frictional resistance.	

FISH Kune-Kune EXERCISE

Slowly loosen the total body

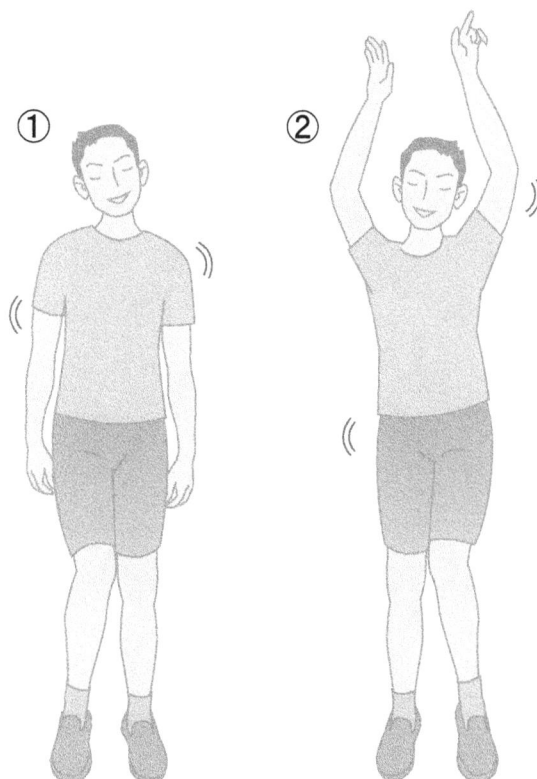

① ②

1) Wiggle your whole body while saying, "kune-kune, kune-kune." Move your spine slowly right and left as if you are a fish swimming in the ocean. Use your entire body. Loosen it completely while saying "kune-kune, kune-kune."
2) Raise both arms and wiggle your whole body again. Once you feel the body is nicely loosened, lower your arms down and keep wiggling.

Japanese Onomatopoeia

kune-kune (*kuu-nay-kuu-nay*)	Describes something that sways or curves gently several times or moves in a wiggling, undulating motion.	

YURU EXERCISE - Basic - STANDING YURU

Fuwa Mozo Underarm

UNDERARM Fuwa Mozo-Mozo EXERCISE

Widely loosen up the underarm area

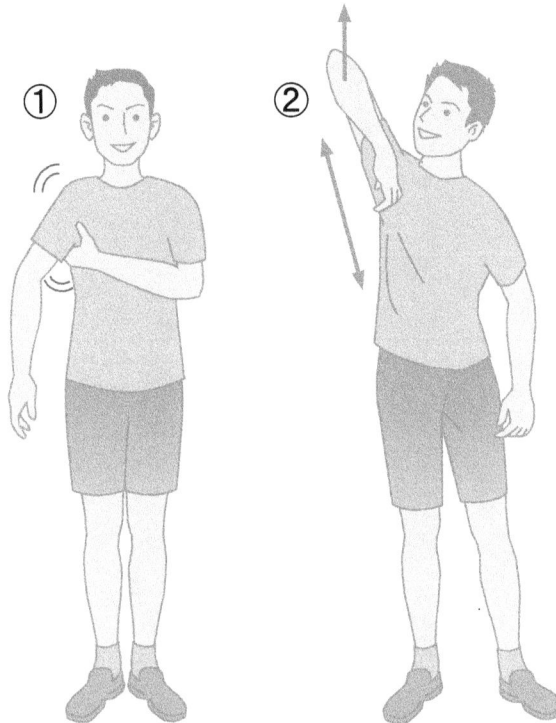

1) Lower your left shoulder. Your left shoulder is just dangling and hanging with no tension. Rub your underarm and the side of your ribs while saying, "Feels good. Feels good." Comfortably rub your underarm while saying, "Feels good. Feels good." Switch arms and repeat.
2) Gently bend your elbow. While saying, "fuwah," open and stretch your left underarm by raising your elbow, upper arm, and shoulder. Switch arms and repeat three times.
3) Wriggle your side torso right and left, up and down to loosen up while saying, "mozo-mozo."

Japanese Onomatopoeia

fuwah	Describes something floating, expanding, soft and fluffy.	
mozo-mozo	Describes something wriggling, wiggling or twisting.	

MORE YURU EXERCISES - Develop each body awareness type -

In the previous pages, I have introduced the basic YURU EXERCISES which are beneficial to all of body awareness types commonly. From here, we will go forward to the specific YURU EXERCISES that are designed for developing and strengthening each body awareness type. Enjoy more YURU EXERCISES!

Develop the center

1. Find the center nearby

The first thing I will teach you is the easiest method. Look around yourself and find something similar to the center. Anything is fine as long as it is a straight vertical line. For example, look at the edge of a column in your house or the line where two walls meet. These lines should be stretched straight up and down. A house or building with a wavy column or one that is built at an angle is probably not very common. Even if you see such a thing, you would feel you don't want to go inside. The fact is that your intuition, "I don't want to go inside," is a very important sensation.

Basically, a column or pillar has to exist as a vertical straight line. Otherwise the house or building cannot maintain its balance. Of course, it is not impossible to build a building with an angled column. However, it is obvious that such a building requires much more intensity and rigidity. Conversely, if a column is built straight, the building can be maintained with minimum intensity because the line matches the vector of gravity.

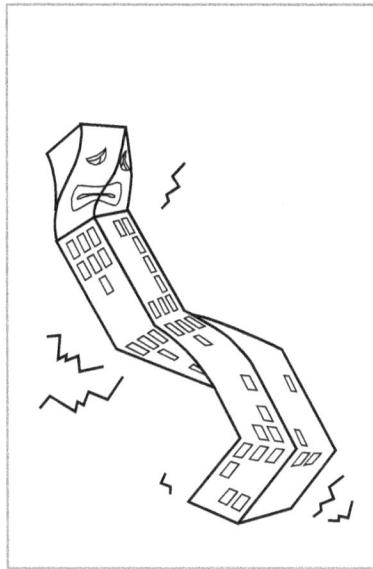

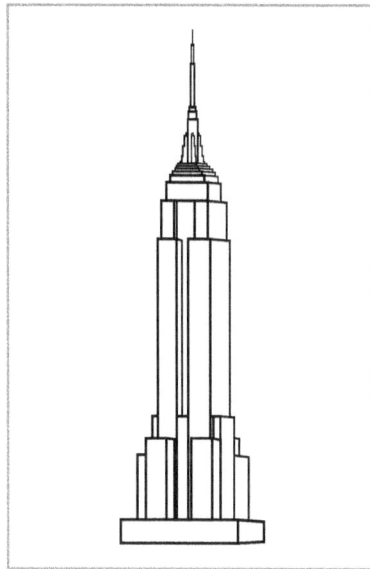

The human body works exactly like this. Therefore, it is important to find your 'environmental center'; the center-like line you see in your environment first to develop the center in your body. Again, anything is fine. The edge of a door, window, or a tall pole you see outside. Try to consciously see something that goes straight up and down. This is the first step of center development training.

2. Feel the center

You should not only look at the center, but also feel it. Use your finger and follow the line twice or three times up and down, up and down. Focus and feel its straightness. Then, place your finger vertically right in front of you. Do you feel something stretching very straight from the middle of your finger? The sensation may not be clear at this point, but you should at least vaguely have this kind of feeling.

Once you obtain that sensation, take it into your body. Where should it go? It goes to the area slightly to the back of the middle of your body, just in front of your spine. Put the straight stretching 'sensation' into that area.

If it is done smoothly, you can do this practice in 30 seconds or less. Use some spare time before starting your regular work or exercise. Do it repeatedly two or three times. Feel the sensation of that center-like line in your body. If you have successfully done this, you will notice your posture has become much better. This 'good posture' is not the one from the stiffness or stillness in your body. It is 'good posture' that looks very natural and you feel very comfortable.

In general, if you are told "Chest up, stand straight." you tend to put a lot of effort into your back muscles. This will make your posture pretty stiff. But if you practice the above method and successfully have the center, you can easily maintain the balance of your body. Your posture will be nice and relaxed as well as very straight. Your center of gravity will be slightly higher than usual. As a result, your eye line is automatically higher. It makes it possible for you to see things from a wider and higher point of view not just physically but also mentally.

Do you feel something has sharpened? Do you feel you can grasp things from a wider and higher point of view? This is the beginning of the center awareness. This training can be done very easily regardless of time and location. Even when you are in a line for a cashier, use a pillar of the store as an environmental center. Let's put the sensation of that centerline into your body.

3. Strengthen the sensation of the center

Once you get used to doing the above training, you can develop the center in your body without pointing your finger vertically. When you don't use your finger, be as close to an environmental center as possible. It should feel easier to do it in this way.

For example, first, stand right in front of a column. Second, get an environmental center visually. Third, put that center into your body. Slowly turn on the spot. This is a tip for better practice. In other words, make a slow anti-clockwise turn along the centerline treating it as an axis. Turn while maintaining the center of your body. This will help you notice that the centerline can be your axis when turning. Your center-like awareness becomes much clearer.

Be mindful about the area around the center in your body. While saying, "Around the center is loosened" gently shake your whole body from the tip of your toes to the head. This step prevents the center from being rigid. This is important because a hard architectural material is usually used as an environmental center in this method which tends to influence people to create rigidity without noticing.

The next step is to gradually walk away from the selected environmental center. When you do this, continue to maintain a good sensation of your center. You should sensitively feel that your arms and legs are moving. This is because of the center axis developed in the center of your body. The parts around the center axis such as your arms or legs can move smoothly and lightly; you can easily feel a pendulum motion.

The environmental center method can even be done just for fun anytime, anywhere. Take it into your daily life and enjoy it. You may find many of your favorite environmental centers. Not just in your house or office but also on the way to your school or workplace; the edge of a tall building, the center of a spiral staircase outside of a building, or the tall chimney of a factory. Set your mind free and find your own environmental center. But don't forget to shake your body to loosen up around the center!

YURU EXERCISE - Develop The Center -

Supah Spine

SPINE CENTERING Supah EXERCISE

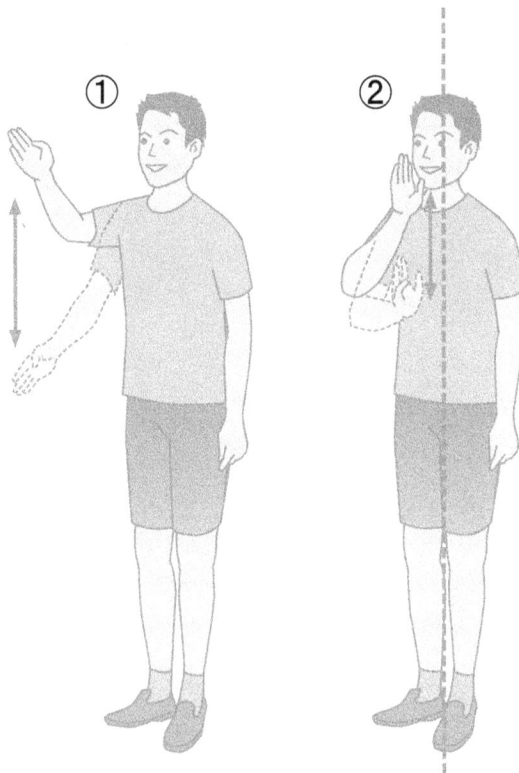

1) Look at a straight vertical line near you. Focus and feel the straightness of that line. While murmuring "How straight it is," follow the line with your left hand, raising and lowering it, up and down, up and down, five or six times.

2) Move your left hand towards you to take the line into your body as if it goes through you right in front of your spine. While saying "supah, supah" follow the line, up and down, up and down, five or six times.

3) Switch arms and repeat 1) and 2).

Japanese Onomatopoeia

supah	Describes something clear or sharp. Describes sharpness when cutting in one motion.	

UNIVERSE LINE CENTERING Supah EXERCISE

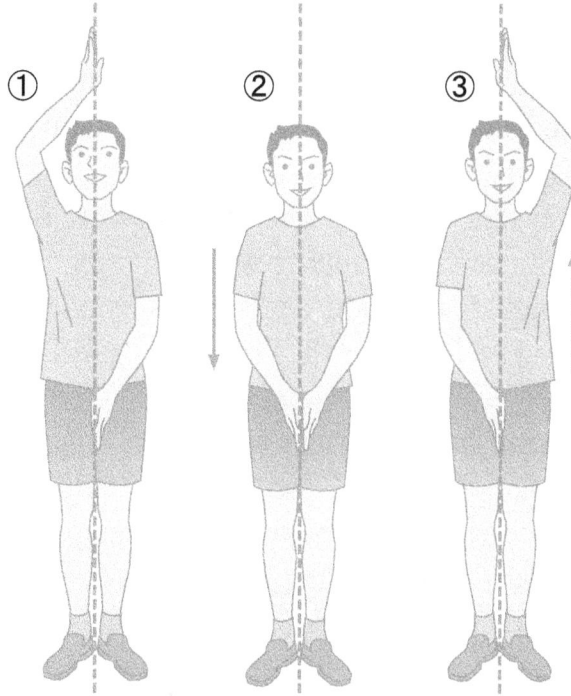

1) Touch your palms and fingers together. Point them toward the center of the earth. While saying "supah," raise and point your right fingers up at the sky while following the line that goes through you right in front of your spine. Look up at the center of sky, then look straight forward.
2) While saying "supah," move your right fingers down the line towards the center of the earth.
3) Switch arms and repeat 1) to 3) three times.

Japanese Onomatopoeia

supah	Describes something clear or sharp.Describes sharpness when cutting in one motion.	

Develop the lower tanden

1. Find and rub the area of the lower tanden

First, find the location of the lower tanden. From the front, it is located in between the navel and the pubic joint. It is the center in the lower abdomen. If you look at yourself from the side, the center of the lower tanden is located in the first third of the torso.

To develop the lower tanden, it is important to locate this spot accurately. Use both hands and rub that area. Keep rubbing while saying, "Feels good. Feels good." You will have a comfortable sensation deep in your abdomen. Once you get this sensation, enjoy that good feeling like "This is nice. It feels so good."

2. Breathe while focusing on the lower tanden

The next step is to focus on your breathing. Inhale through your nose. Imagine the fresh air is naturally going all the way down to your lower tanden. Then, slowly exhale. Exhale while maintaining the fulfillment sensation in the lower tanden. When you breathe out, you can even use Japanese onomatopoeia, "poko (belly out)." This helps to practice effectively.

Let's do it again. First, inhale deeply. As you exhale only one third of the breath, say "poko" (belly out). Keep exhaling another one third of the breath, while saying "peko" (belly in). Keep exhaling the last third of the breath, while saying "pokooo" (belly out). Repeat several times. Notice that the fulfillment sensation in your lower tanden becomes stronger and stronger with each practice. (See the instruction below "ABDOMEN Poko Peko Pokooo EXERCISE")

Some breathing exercises require you to count a certain number of times in your mind during the practice. However, counting is not good for creating the lower tanden. Because when you count, your awareness tends to be interrupted at each count. This will make it difficult for you to have the sense of fulfillment and stability that is needed to develop the lower tanden. So, go at your own pace. Slower breathing is always better. But it is important that you do not feel uncomfortable with this practice. The key for this exercise is to practice at your own pace and speed. Do not push yourself.

If you have not done any breathing exercises or never thought about the lower tanden, this exercise would work well even if you only do it three times. Again, you do not need to push yourself. It is nice to be motivated like, "OK, I will create the best lower tanden I can!" However, none of the YURU EXERCISES require hard work. Working too hard makes your body inflexible and you'll tend to put in too much effort and energy. This will produce bad results.

When your lower tanden is in good shape, you will gain great benefits such as 'calmness,' 'confidence,' and an 'unflappable attitude.' However, if you create the lower tanden in an inflexible body, you will likely be a person who is 'confident but stiff and cold,' or 'composed but with no compassion for the sorrow of others.' This kind of person is ok by himself but very boring and bothersome socially. Not just for the lower tanden, but also for all other training methods to develop the body awareness, it is very important not to practice too hard but to focus on loosening your body.

YURU EXERCISE - Develop The Lower Tanden -

Fuwa Abs Back

LOWER ABDOMEN Fuwa & LOWER BACK AND HIP Fuwa EXERCISE

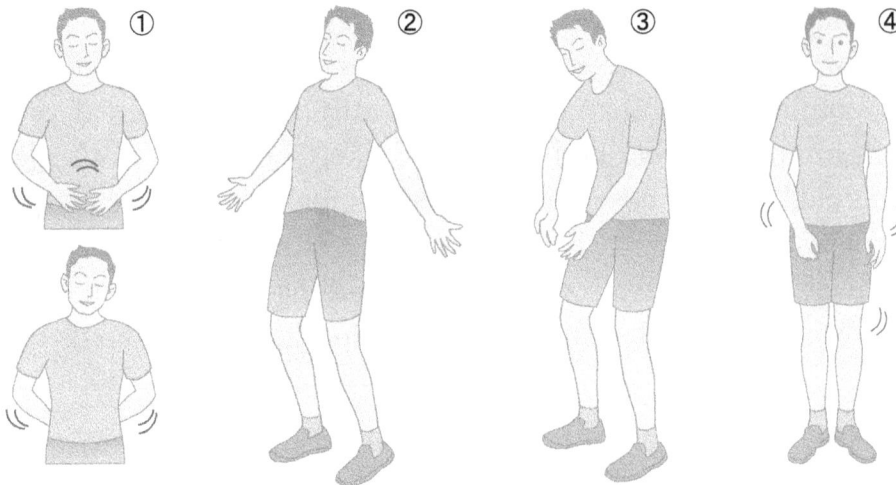

1) Rub your lower abdomen gently and comfortably with both hands while saying, "Feels good. Feels good." Next, rub your lower back while saying, "Feels good. Feels good."
2) Open and stretch your lower abdomen while saying "fuwah."
3) Open and stretch your hips and lower back while saying "fuwah." Repeat 2) and 3) three times.
4) Wriggle your lower abdomen and hips right and left, right and left while saying "mozo-mozo, mozo-mozo." Imagine those parts are totally loosened.

Note: It may sound a little difficult to have the sensation where you have relaxed and opened your hips and lower back. The key point, before you start this exercise, is to focus on the area to be loosened by shaking your hips lightly. When you loosen your hips and lower back, think that all of the muscles around your lumbar spine are separated and relaxed.

Japanese Onomatopoeia

| fuwah | Describes something soft, fluffy, floating and expanding. | |
| mozo-mozo | Describes something wriggling, wiggling or twisting. | |

ABDOMEN Poko Peko Pokooo EXERCISE

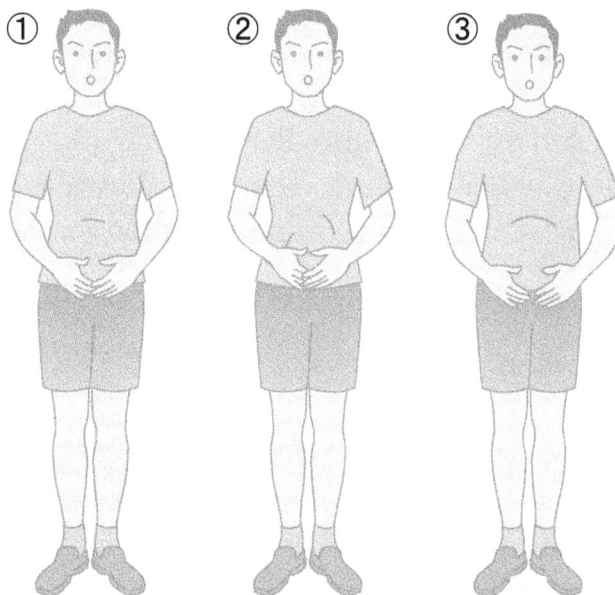

1) Use both hands and rub your lower abdomen while saying, "Feels good. Feels good."
2) Exhale deeply. Then, deeply inhale through your nose. Your chest expands. As you exhale the first third of the breath, say "poko." Your lower belly is out.
3) Keep exhaling the next third of the breath, while saying "peko." Your lower belly is in.
4) Keep exhaling the last of the breath, while saying "pokooo." Your lower belly is out. Repeat 2) to 4) three times.

Japanese Onomatopoeia

poko/pokooo	Describes something expanded. Convex.	
peko	Describes something indented. Concave.	

Develop the middle tanden

1. Rub and loosen your entire chest

First, gently rub your entire chest well. Not just for the middle tanden but also for all other body awareness types, it is important to loosen and relax the target area in advance. In addition to this, gently rub the whole chest area and loosen it to practice the middle tanden training. This will allow you to create the relaxed awareness in an appropriate way and location. The Chest Fuwa & Back Fuwa Exercise explained below is the most appropriate training method for the start of creating the middle tanden.

2. Tap your middle tanden

The center of the middle tanden is located at the level of the lower third of the breastbone. There is an easy way to determine its location. Place the first joint (the biggest joint attached to your palm) of your pinky on the bottom edge of your breastbone. From that point to the higher point where your index finger touches — that is the center area of the middle tanden.

First, look at the illustration below. Shape your hand as if you were holding a grapefruit or softball. This shape is called the Five Fingers Energy. Maintain this shape and tap the center of the middle tanden.

In the Five Fingers Energy, there is a space that you can put an imaginary ball. That ball is the shape of the middle tanden. You are supposed to put the ball into your chest by tapping your chest with the Five Fingers Energy. However, please note that this practice is a strong stimulus. Do not tap too much. Usually tapping six times or at most 10 times a day is good enough.

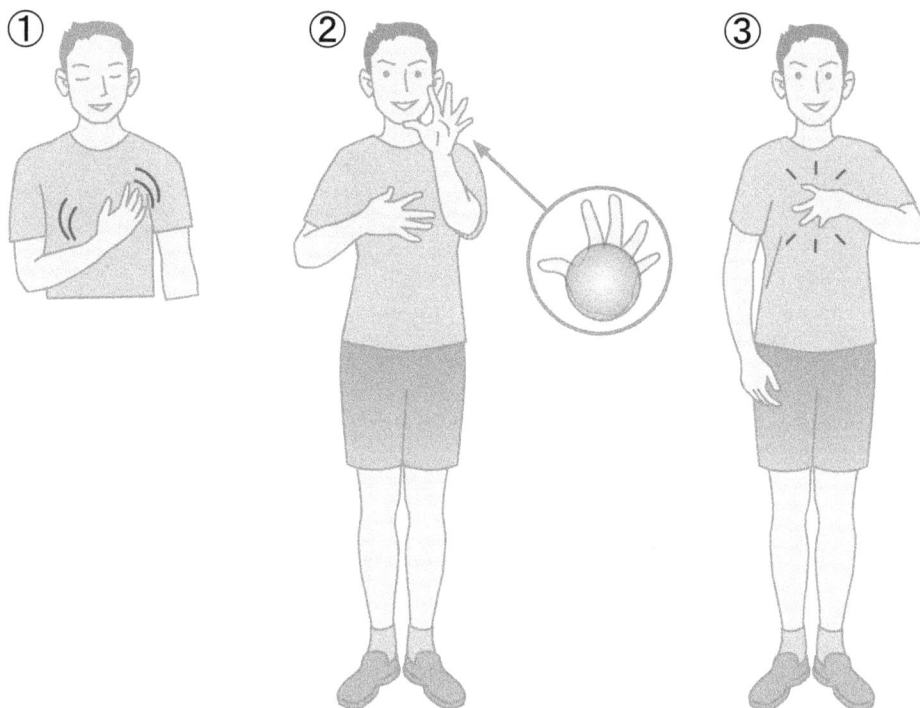

It is highly recommended that you develop the middle tanden together with the lower tanden. The middle tanden is the center where hot energies gather. Having only the middle tanden means you have nothing to control the hot energies. When well controlled, these hot energies can work for 'great passion,' 'cherishing or holding high esteem for others,' or 'loving others with great care.' However, if the middle tanden is out of control, you would tend to generate too much excitement, your love for others may become excessive or aberrational, or you would tend to be upset or lose your temper easily. If your test score in Chapter 3 shows that you have a strong lower tanden but not much for the middle tanden, then focusing on the training for the middle tanden would be good for you.

Also please keep in mind that the shape of the Five Fingers Energy has an important meaning. You can put hot energies properly into the space created by your fingers in this shape. Thus, please do not make a fist to tap your chest. Tapping your chest with your fist will work to heat your chest. But you will not have a clear image or shape of the middle tanden. Without its clear image, there is a risk that the hot energies would not stay in your middle tanden but would spread out to your head or other areas in your body.

YURU EXERCISE - Develop The Middle Tanden -

Fuwa Chest Back

CHEST Fuwa & BACK Fuwa EXERCISE

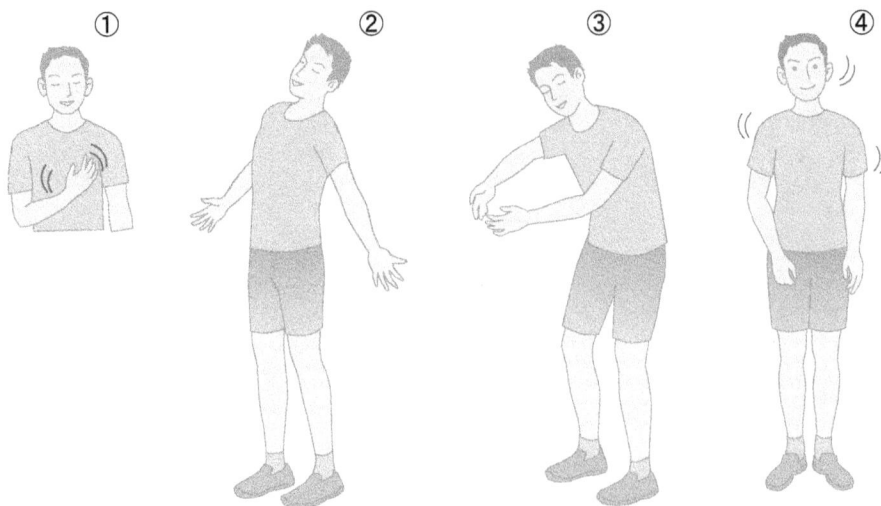

1) Rub your whole chest gently while saying, "Feels good. Feels good."
2) Open your chest wide by pulling back your shoulders and arms gently and softly, while saying, "fuwah."
3) Open your back wide, gently bringing your arms forward, saying, "fuwah." Repeat 2) and 3) several times.
4) Wriggle your chest and back right and left, up and down. Say, "mozo-mozo." Imagine your chest and back are totally loosened. Inside your body is completely relaxed, too.

Note: Release all the tension in your upper torso. When you open your chest, lean back on a large imaginary balloon. When you open your back, gently hug another large balloon in front of you. "Open the back" and "open the chest" do not simply mean to expand or stretch your back and chest. You should focus on inside your body. Opening your back and chest will create more space between each body part. Imagine that each muscle, bone structure, and cell in your chest and back are totally loosened and expanded.

Japanese Onomatopoeia

fuwah	Describes something soft, fluffy, floating and expanding.	
mozo-mozo	Describes something wriggling, wiggling or twisting.	

CHEST FIVE FINGERS ENERGY EXERCISE

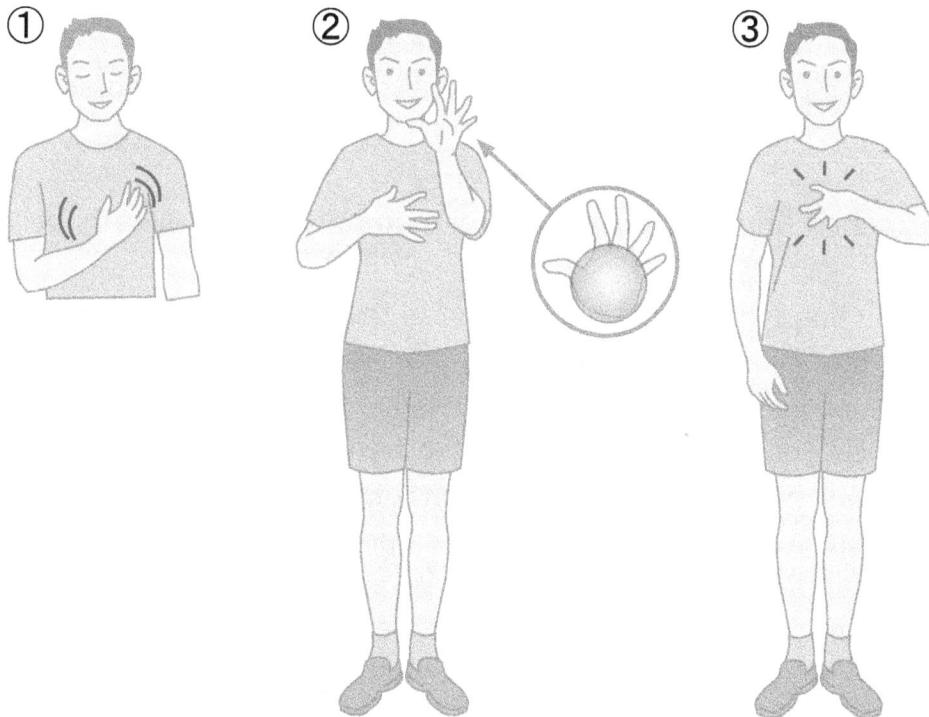

1) Rub your chest with your left hand while saying, "Feels good. Feels good." Switch arms and repeat. Use both hands and keep rubbing while saying, "Feels good. Feels good."
2) Open your left fingers and make a space on your palm. The space should be as big as a grapefruit or softball.
3) Maintain this shape and place your fingers on your lower chest. Gently tap your chest six times. Imagine you are sending a warm-hearted message or courage into the center of your chest.
4) Switch arms and repeat.

Develop the arch

1. Rub your chest

The arch is the body awareness type that is the easiest to practice among the seven awareness types. Gently rub your chest well and feel yourself warm and comfortable.

2. Create arched line awareness between you and another person

Place your dominant hand on the center of the middle tanden. Move your hand by following the imaginary gentle arched line from you to another person who is actually there or while imagining that person. The movement of your hand will guide to connect you and the person with the arched line.

The key point here is to put your emotions or words into that movement. For example, if you are antisocial, afraid of meeting people, or if you feel that somebody rejects you, then try this. Before meeting with another person, draw an imaginary arch while saying quietly "I would like to have empathy for you. Please have empathy for me, too." While following the line of the arch with your hand, think about giving and receiving such words. It will be more effective than simply drawing the line silently. If you have a weak middle tanden, it's good to practice the middle tanden training first, then try the arch training. However, if your lower tanden has not been developed yet, I recommend you don't do the middle tanden training.

Similar to the other body awareness types, the arch training needs to be done gradually, little by little. This applies to not just the body awareness training but also to any other training, including muscle training. If you become rapidly enthusiastic about one thing, even if it is a lesson in foreign language conversation, you would likely be overwhelmed. If it is muscle training, you might hurt your muscles. If it is stretching, you could hurt your joints or tendons. That is why you do not need to practice the arch training 20 or 30 times from the beginning. For beginners, practicing six times a day would be sufficient. You can gradually increase the number of practices, but I would say 20 times a day is maximum. (Here, one time means one round - following the arch to/from another person.)

More practically, the arch can be practiced in a real world situation. As mentioned in Chapter 2, if you are a sales person, you can say quietly "I am going to talk to you about something important. Please listen to me." before greeting a customer. Then follow the imaginary arched line four to six times using your finger. You can talk to the other person more freely and comfortably than usual. Even if a topic is complicated or difficult, unnecessary tension or doubts can be avoided. The conversation will likely go frankly and smoothly.

This is just an aside, but a great business is not something where you focus on your own benefit or profit. It is something where you value the other person's benefit or profit as well. As people used to say, the essence of business lies in 'sincerity' and 'empathy.' The arch creates a great affinity in your circumstances. Once it is there, you and others can find a good touch point in each other and will have a long-term relationship.

YURU EXERCISE - Develop The Arch -

CHEST TO CHEST EMPATHY EXERCISE

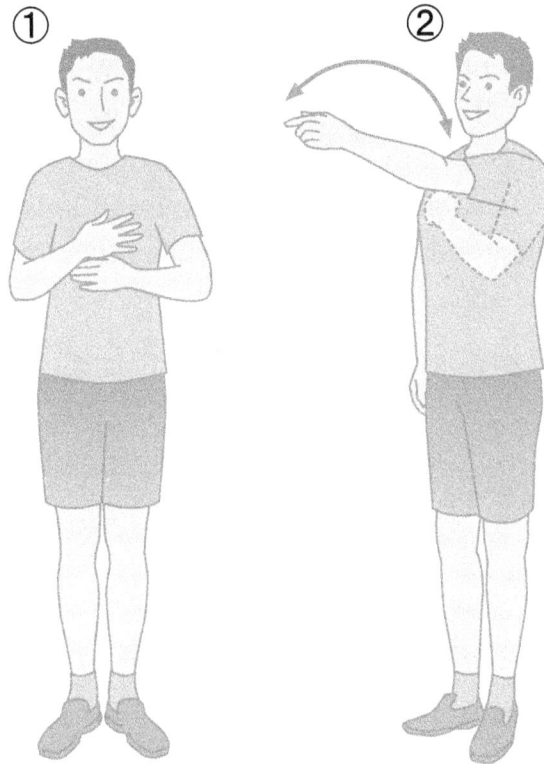

1) Gently rub your chest while saying, "Feels good. Feels good." Switch hands and repeat. Use both hands and keep rubbing your chest while saying, "Feels good. Feels good."
2) Think of the person with whom you wish to share empathy. Imagine that the center of your chest and the center of that person's chest are connected with the arched line. Think of the line that goes from the center of your chest to the center of the other person's chest. Next, think of the line that returns from the center of the other person's chest to the center of your chest. Put your mind and the emotion of empathy into the movement of this arch practice.
3) To the person with whom you wish to have empathy, follow the arch for two or three rounds while saying, "I would like to have empathy with you. I would like you to have empathy with me. I wish to have empathy with you. I wish you to have empathy with me, too. I would like to have empathy with you. I would like you to have empathy with me. I wish to have empathy with you. I wish you to have empathy with me, too. I wish we will have empathy with each other. I wish we will have empathy with each other."

Develop the vest

1. Rub your vest lines

As you can see in the illustration below, the vest lines draw curves that go through the following points; the middle of sternoclavicular and acromioclavicular joints (in other words, the middle of the collarbone), the nipples, and go towards the underarms. You can make sure of the points on your underarms by gently dropping down your arms and placing your four fingers right below the underarms. The vest lines go through the points where your pinky touches. On the back side of the torso, the vest lines go through the following points; the middle of the shoulder blades and spine, the edges of the trapezius muscles, and come back to the middle of the collarbone.

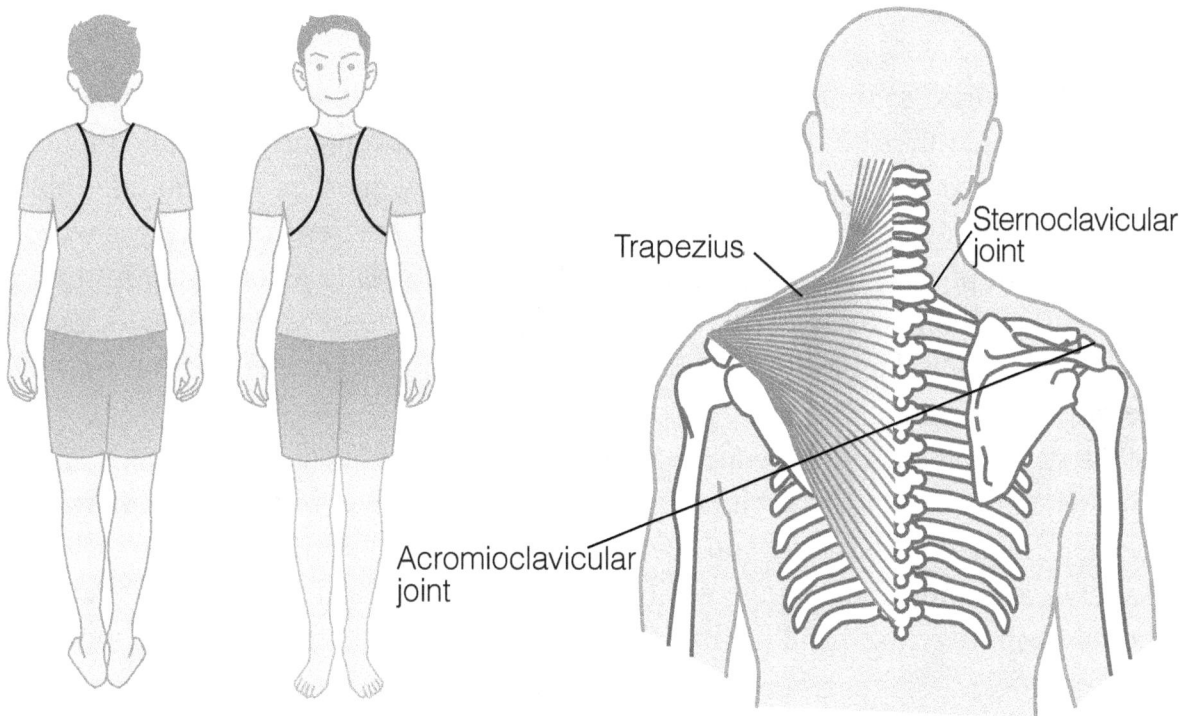

As explained, the vest lines go around your shoulders. Use your fingers and rub these lines well. Make sure to rub both sides. I know you probably cannot reach the backside. Ask a family member or a friend to rub the unreachable areas. If no one is available to help you, use an object such as the corner of a column. This is the first step of the vest training.

The awareness of the vest can be made stronger by rubbing the lines. Even just rubbing will bring you some benefits. After you rubbed the lines well, do you feel something different? Do you feel that the rubbed areas are kind of warm and loosened? Your shoulders and back are supposed to be warm and loosened, too. You should feel a relaxed sensation in your underarms.

Once the entire vest lines become warm and loosened, change your focus onto your shoulders and arms. Do you feel the difference before and after rubbing the lines? You probably used to feel your shoulders and arms were tight and tense. Do you feel that the bases of both your arms used to be located more to the outside?

Of course the locations of your shoulder joints never change, even after you have rubbed the vest lines. However now you probably feel like the shoulder joints have deepened and extended up to the vest lines. Enjoy this sensation. This is the very first benefit from the vest.

As explained in the previous chapter, the vest will allow you to use your arms from far inside the shoulder blades. Although the movement from the ribs is not well recognized even in the sports world yet, the movement of the shoulder blades is now attracting attention. In Japan, the existence of the vest has been regarded as extremely important in the world of swordplay. The master swordsmen in the Edo period all used this vest in their swordplay. I am sure that the vest will be focused on by the sports world as well in the near future as a factor that enables and improves the movement of the ribs and shoulder blades.

Now, let's focus on the entire torso before and after rubbing your vest lines. I think your torso was pretty tight and inflexible before rubbing. But after rubbing the vest lines, do you think you feel more comfortable with your torso? Can you make various movements quite easily? Especially the areas around your shoulders should be more relaxed and flexible. You might even feel you can breathe more easily.

2. Move your body by following the vest lines

Once your vest awareness has increased, move your body in the following order, first the shoulders, then the chest, the underarms, the back, and finally returning to your shoulders. This is the second step of the vest training. The point here is you should not put too much effort into this practice. It is good to start with your shoulder areas while saying "kururi(kuu-ruu-ri), kururi(kuu-ruu-ri)." "kururi" is a Japanese onomatopoeia describing rolling, rotating or spinning.

First, roll your shoulders from back to front while saying "kururi, kururi." Once your shoulder areas become loosened, use its motion memory to rotate your ribs from back to front. Repeat it for a while.

How do you feel? I think you strongly feel that your shoulder joints are now more deeply expanded towards the inside. When you first noticed the vest lines by rubbing them, you might have had an awareness of only the surface of your body. But after you moved your body following the vest lines, you should have a stronger awareness from inside your body and feel more relaxed. Your torso should be more flexible. You may feel you are kind of moving even if you are still. Some people may be able to breathe much easier and feel greater comfort.

YURU EXERCISE - Develop The Vest -

Kururi Shoulder Ribs
-Forward-

SHOULDER Kururi RIBS Kururi FORWARD ROLLING EXERCISE

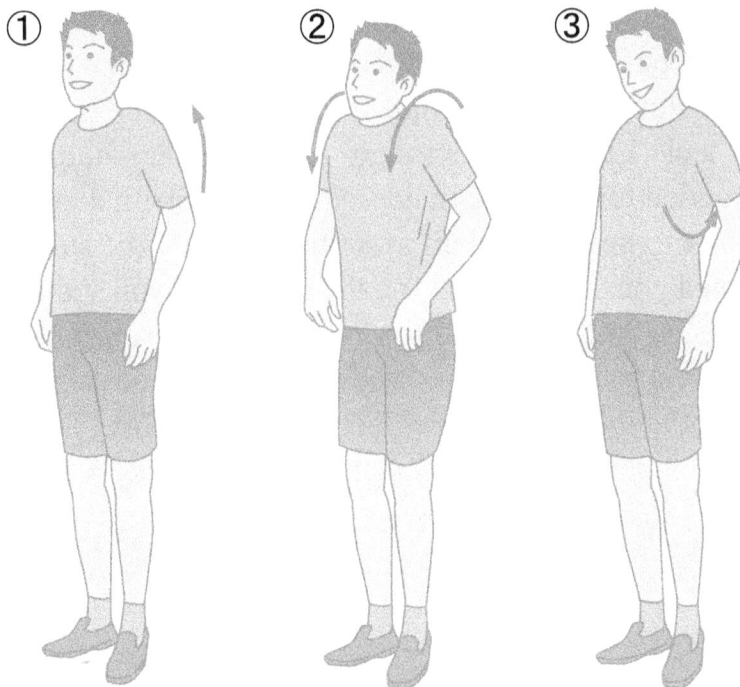

1) Slightly lower your left shoulder. Rub your left shoulder while saying, "Feels good. Feels good." Switch arms and lower your right shoulder. Rub your right shoulder while saying, "Feels good. Feels good."

2) Roll your shoulders from back to front while saying "kururi, kururi." Imagine that your shoulders are becoming more loosened and relaxed with each rotation.

3) In the same rhythm, use the above motion memory, and together with your shoulders, roll your ribs from back to front while saying "kururi, kururi." Your ribs should become more loosened and relaxed with each rotation. Roll your shoulders, saying, "kururi, kururi." Roll your ribs saying, "kururi, kururi."

Japanese Onomatopoeia

kururi (kuu-ruu-ri)	Describes rolling, rotating, or spinning.	

SHOULDER Kururi RIBS Kururi BACKWARD ROLLING EXERCISE

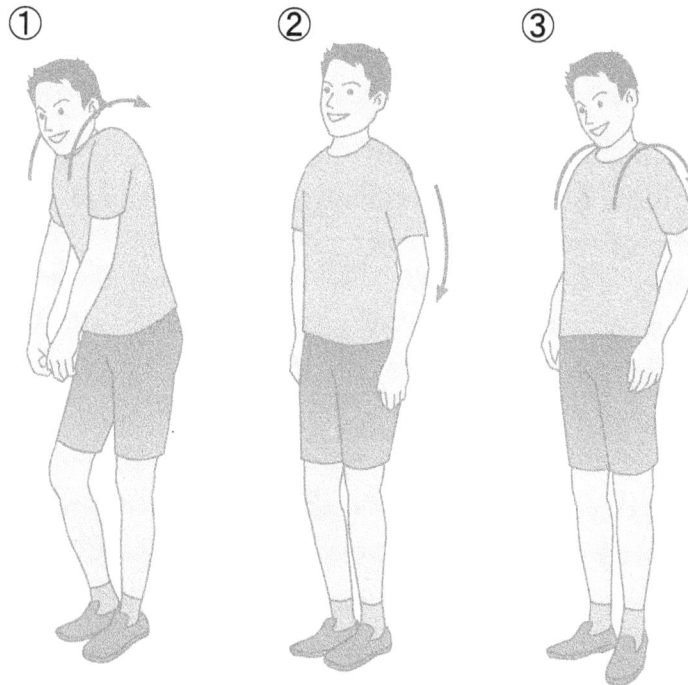

① ② ③

1) Slightly lower your left shoulder. Rub your left shoulder while saying, "Feels good. Feels good." Switch arms and lower your right shoulder. Rub your right shoulder while saying, "Feels good. Feels good." Roll your shoulders from front to back while saying "kururi, kururi." Imagine that your shoulders are becoming more loosened and relaxed with each rotation.

2) In the same rhythm, use the above motion memory, and together with your shoulder, roll your ribs front to back while saying "kururi, kururi." Your ribs should become more loosened and relaxed with each rotation. Roll your shoulders saying, "kururi, kururi." Roll your ribs saying, "kururi, kururi."

Japanese Onomatopoeia

kururi (kuu-ruu-ri)	Describes rolling, rotating, or spinning.	

Develop the uratenshi (back push)

1. Rub your uratenshi

First determine the location of the uratenshi. Touch the keypoints on both legs:

Point A: The bottom of your buttocks (the core of the uratenshi)
Point B: The back side of your knees
Point C: The middle of the line connecting from A and B
Point D: The center level of your buttocks

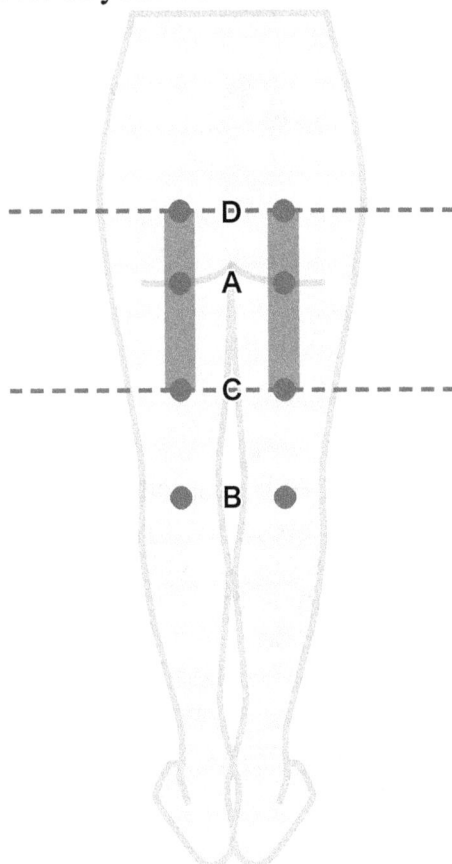

Second, connect C and D. The uratenshi is the awareness of the strip-like shapes located on those lines. Once you understand the location, rub that part well and focus your mind on the uratenshi.

Let's try the ONE KNEE REST BACK THIGH Suri-Suri EXERCISE (see detailed instructions below). Rub your left uratenshi. Keep rubbing until the line of your uratenshi gets warm. Then, walk at least five or six steps.

How did you feel? Did you feel something like a strip or line on your left back thigh? The reason why you feel this is because your hamstrings and gluteus maximus muscles are working well centering your hip joints. When you are walking forward and supporting your weight on your left leg, your body should move strongly and smoothly. You should walk evenly with a relatively higher center of gravity.

Once you feel these sensations, switch legs and rub your right uratenshi well. Just like you did for your left side, rub your right back thigh well. Then, walk forward five to six steps.

How did you feel? You should have had a feeling that you could go forward vigorously. From a technical point of view, if you stimulate your uratenshi appropriately, the movement of your first and second steps becomes faster. In other words, your motive force is completely different compared with before and after rubbing. Hamstrings and the gluteus are special muscles - accelerative muscles - to spur you to move forward. If you have a strong awareness and it is activated in your hamstrings and gluteus, your motive force will increase dramatically. If you have the sensation of the strip or line on the uratenshi area that is the same area of the hamstrings and gluteus, it would be proof that those muscles are well used centering your hip joints.

The very first step to develop the uratenshi is to rub that area on both sides very well. The more you rub, the more benefits you gain. You can rub anytime. At the same time, rubbing each side up to 30 times in total each day would be good enough.

YURU EXERCISE - Develop The Uratenshi -

Ussu Suri Thigh

Ussu Suri-Suri EXERCISE

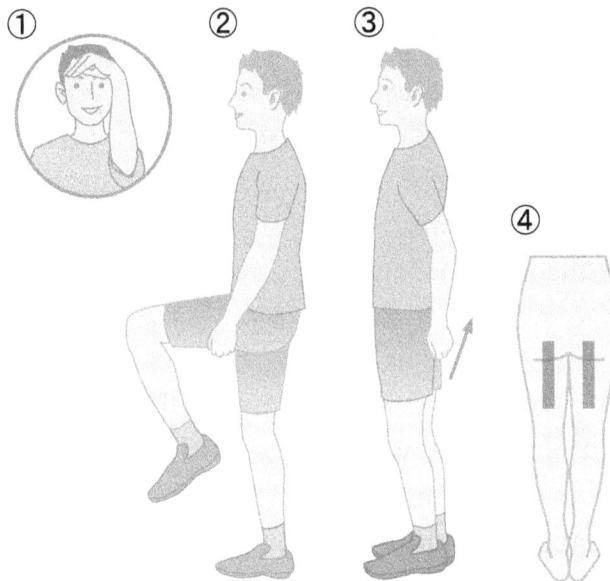

① ② ③

④

1) While saying, "Ussu!" shape your left hand like the bill of a cap and place it on your forehead. Slightly and gently bend your fingertips. All your left fingers are still touching together. Bend the base joints of your left fingers. Your wrist should also be bent at a 90° angle.
2) Lower your left hand all the way down while maintaining the shape of your left hand. Raise your left thigh until it is parallel to the floor. Put your left hand under the center of your back thigh.
3) While saying, "suri, suri," strongly rub your left upper thigh and lower buttocks. Lower your leg down to the floor. Repeat several times until the uratenshi becomes warm. Switch sides and repeat several times. Stand straight naturally. If you do not feel balanced, repeat the above until you have the same sensation in both legs. Once you feel nice and evenly balanced, the exercise is done.

Note: "Ussu" is an informal Japanese greeting similar to "Hi!" or "Hey!" It is mostly used by men. Even if you are non-Japanese or female; try saying "Ussu!" like a karate player. Say it as a joke. Saying "Ussu!" sends your spirit and energy into your hands. This will allow you to rub your uratenshi strong enough. Remember, laughing is important for YURU EXERCISES. The more you laugh, the more your body and mind become relaxed, loosened, and healthier.

This exercise stimulates your uratenshi, the strip-shaped awareness located on your lower buttocks and upper back thighs. By stimulating or focusing on this area, you will be able to swing your femurs (thighbones) smoothly.

Japanese Onomatopoeia

suri-suri	Describes nuzzling, snuggling or rubbing.	

ONE KNEE REST BACK THIGH Suri-Suri EXERCISE

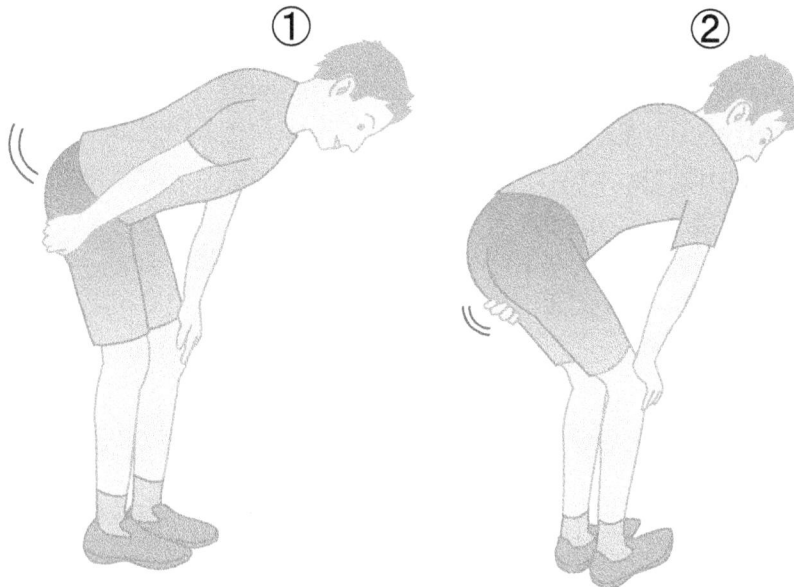

1) Stand straight and open your legs slightly narrower than your hip width distance. While sticking out your buttocks, gently put your hands on your knees. While putting your weight on your left hand, touch your buttocks and the upper part of your right back thigh (the line of the uratenshi) with your right hand. Release all tension in your back and hips. Your left arm is naturally stretched and supporting your torso. Stay in this position.

2) Rub the backside of your right thigh (the right uratenshi) while saying, "Feels good. Feels good." Rub it even stronger while whispering, "Right here. Suri-suri." Keep rubbing stronger and stronger while saying, "Right here. Suri-suri."

3) Switch arms and legs. Repeat several times.

Japanese Onomatopoeia

suri-suri	Describes nuzzling, snuggling or rubbing.	

Develop the laser

1. Press the laser starting point

Similar to the lower tanden, make sure you find the key location first. Use the middle finger of your right hand; gently press several times on the point that is at the mid-point between your navel and your pubic joint. Focus on your sacrum that is located right behind the lower tanden. The laser is the line awareness that starts and stretches from the sacrum.

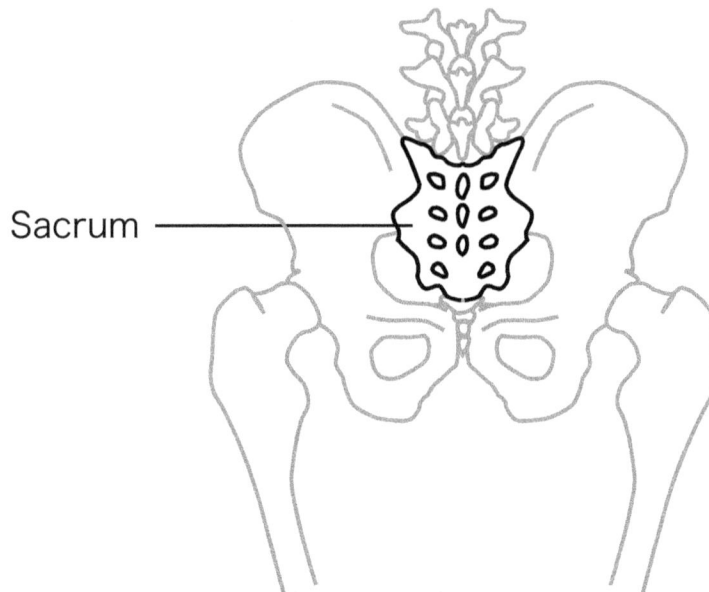

Sacrum

Next, use your left thumb and press the sacrum from your back. This means that you should use both hands to press your lower tanden and sacrum to connect the awareness back and forth, created between your fingers. Press many times and focus on the awareness connecting your left thumb and right middle finger.

2. Extend your laser

Once you have created the awareness of the laser starting point, point your right index finger forward. Think that the line from the sacrum stretches far forward. If you are in a room, extend your line awareness to the very end of the wall. If you are in a hallway, extend your line awareness to the far end of the hallway. Stretch the line all way to the most distant end point that you can see. Then, walk forward following that line awareness.

How did you feel? Did you feel you could walk very straight? You might have felt the existence of an invisible guideline to walk. It should be created by your stretched line awareness. This is the benefit that you can recognize most easily. Because of this awareness, you will be directly connected to your target. This will smoothly strengthen the vector or orbit towards your target.

In Japan, there is an expression used when talking about a soul-mate, [watashi wa ano hito to akai ito de tsunagatte iru] ("I am connected to him/her with a red thread"). Similar to this, if you develop the laser, you will have a feeling that you are tightly connected with others.

Another benefit that you gain from the laser is your walking style will be more stable. You will not be wobbly but can walk very smoothly. This is proof that you are not wasting power on your outer muscles. If you put too much power on your outer muscles, you would tend to walk heavily and awkwardly. However, the laser can loosen your body. It also affects the uratenshi and the center. The laser makes them work more effectively.

If you develop the laser, you can also apply it to a target at your workplace (something other than an object or person).

3. Use your laser at work

For example, set a target at your workplace. First, put your targeted thing or task in front of you. The thing or task may sound too abstract; they actually vary depending on the person. You can think about something that can be a symbol of your target. Put it in front of you. If you are sales person, it could be a customer's folder or computer. If you are a cook, it could be cooking ingredients or a cooking utensil. If you are an engineer or mechanic, it could be a machine. Anything is fine. Think of something that can be a symbol of your 'job target' and set a sight on the center of your 'job target' using your laser.

Press your sacrum with your left thumb. Place your right index finger on your lower tanden. Point your right index finger towards your target. This helps you set your laser, aiming it accurately and effectively. You can even say, "pishii." This is another Japanese onomatopoeia describing something sharp, clear or straight.

Even more effective is to put words and emotions into your awareness. "This work is very important. But it is tough. I may feel like giving up, but I can never escape from my work. I can achieve my target." This way combines your emotion or motivation and your actual words such as "I can do it!" and puts them into your laser.

The other thing is, when you talk to somebody about something important, connect your laser that comes from the center of yourself to the center of that person. This will create a strict association between you and the target person like "This topic is so significant that we cannot avoid discussing it." However, this could also create unnecessary tension as well. If that happens, the basic YURU EXERCISES can help. The laser actually works best when your body and mind are nicely loosened − and even better is creating the arch above the laser. You can have a strong relationship with others like, "A steady relationship is necessary to successfully complete this work." At the same time, friendly emotion and affinity will be created as well without having a strained relationship.

Using the laser and the arch allows you to succeed even with difficult negotiations at work. You will not feel like escaping or avoiding conversations with others. Instead, you will be able to proceed with your negotiations while affinity is maintained. Especially for human relationships, combining the laser and the arch can be very effective.

SACRUM LASER LINE Pishii EXERCISE

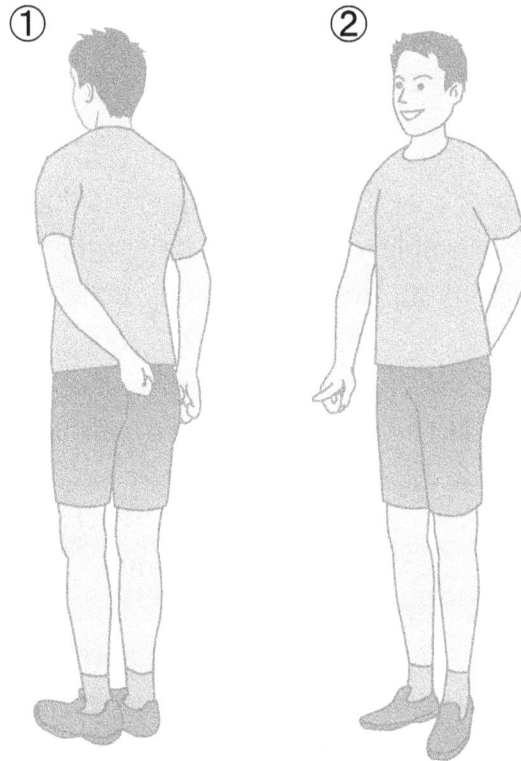

① ②

1) Press the center of your sacrum (the back side of your body) with your left thumb while saying, "pishii." Imagine that your laser starts from your sacrum and stretches through the center of your lower tanden, and extends straight forward.
2) In order to strengthen the line and stretch it further, place your right index finger in front of your lower tanden. While saying, "pishii" in one exhalation, point your right index finger forward.
3) Switch arms and repeat.

Japanese Onomatopoeia

pishii	Describing something sharp, clear, disciplined or straight.	

Chapter 5

Examples of the Benefits of the YURU EXERCISES to Develop Body Awareness

The benefits of the YURU EXERCISES to develop body awareness are enormous. I have heard many of them from my students or at my workshop. At last, I would like to share some examples with you. I hope other people's experiences will help you discover and enjoy your developing body awareness.

Note: When you practice the YURU EXERCISES, you can get benefits instantly in some cases. In other cases, it will take time and require constant practice before realizing the benefits. For example, when you practice your golf swing, you might feel benefits immediately after doing the WRIST Pura-Pura EXERCISE and other exercises that develop the vest. Another example is practicing the exercises to develop the arch before speaking in front of an audience at a conference or visiting customers for your business. On the other hand, it may take time to see the benefits of the center or the lower tanden for someone who is short tempered or someone who gets in trouble easily. Those people may need several months of training before feeling like "I am strong and can deal with difficulties better," or "I can deal with problems very calmly." The amount of benefit and the required period of practice will vary among different individuals.

Center
James: Company director

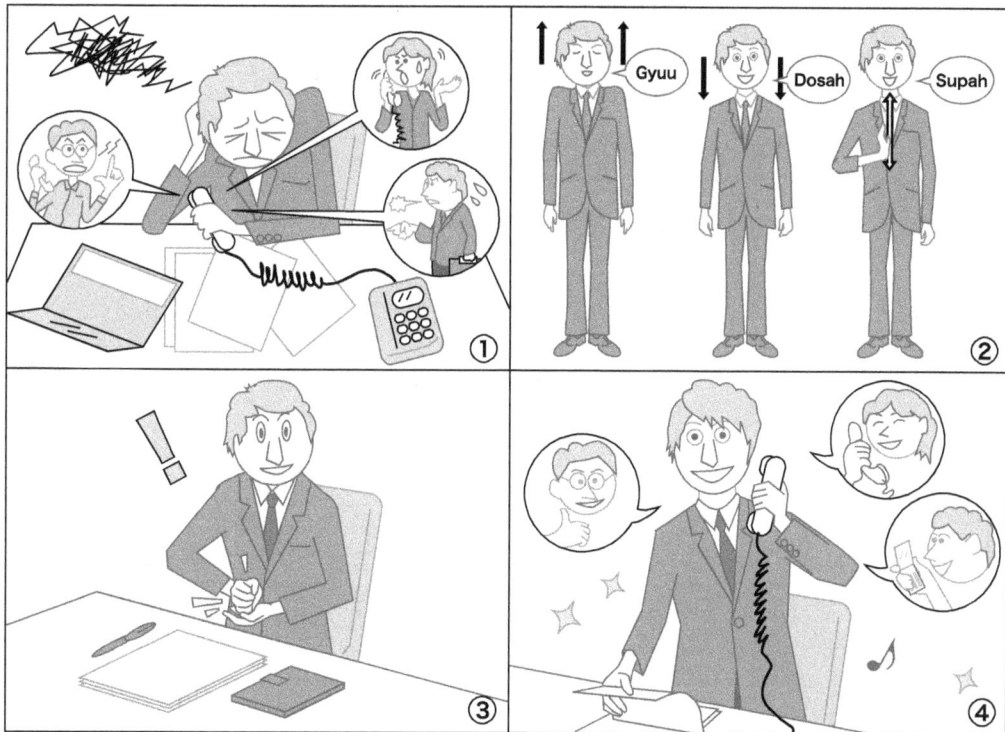

James' project was a full of problems. Nothing was working properly. He received many claims and complaints from his clients and subordinates almost every day. He was totally exhausted. His mind was completely unbalanced. He was even losing his confidence in directing his project.

But, CENTER!! He remembered the center and focused on it. "Gyuu," "dosah," "supah," "See things from a wider and higher point of view." He reminded himself.

His spine straightened. A balanced posture made his mind clear, centered, and grounded. He could rethink each problem one by one. What's more important? What's less important? What's the first thing to do? What's the right thing to do? He could recognize and organize his issues well. He focused on the most important issue and didn't worry about minor issues. He could also feel more generous to others and noticed their many good points and strengths. Soon he could handle and lead his project in a better way.

Lower Tanden
Daniel: Department manager

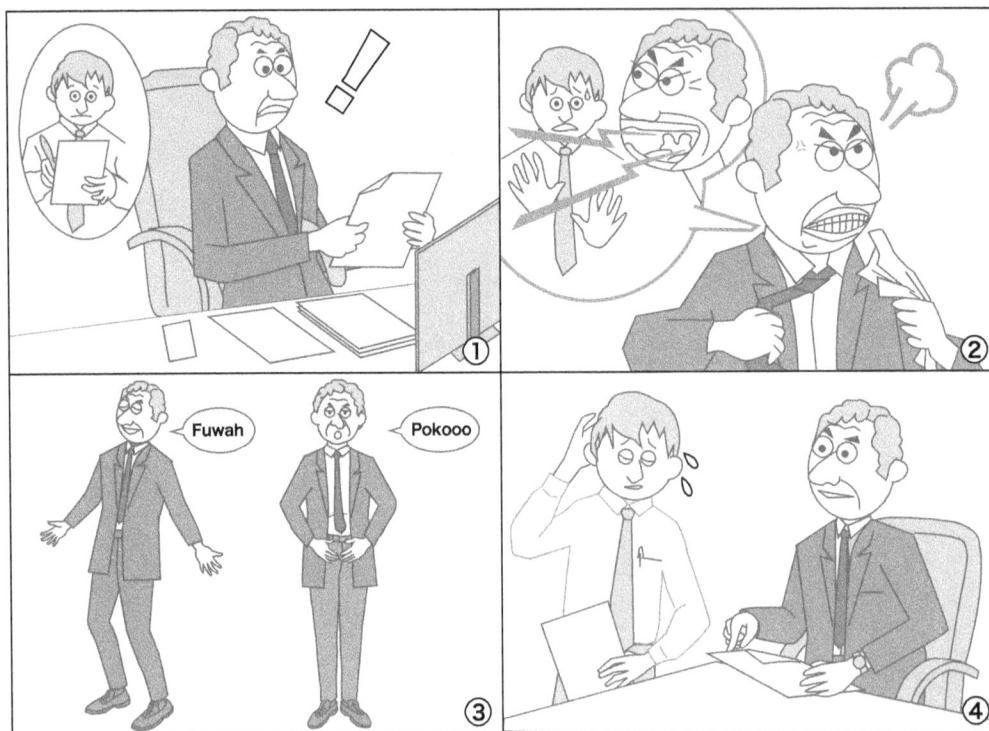

Daniel often gets mad and frustrated with mistakes made by his subordinates. One day, he asked John to prepare presentation documents to be used in the following week. When he checked the documents, he noticed many mistakes. "Give me a break! Not again!" He wanted to call John immediately and yell at him to make him realize how careless he was. Daniel felt anger swelling inside. He was almost losing his temper.

"No, I shouldn't be like this." He focused his lower tanden. To make himself calm down, he tried the LOWER ABDOMEN Fuwa & LOWER BACK AND HIP Fuwa EXERCISE and the ABDOMEN Poko Peko Pokooo EXERCISE. He noticed that his anger became much less as he calmed down.

When John came to his office, Daniel stayed calm and pointed out his mistakes gently and rationally. John felt something was different from usual. In a better atmosphere, he could accept Daniel's points. John seemed to open his mind and could understand Daniel's feedback with more respect.

Middle Tanden
Sandra: Elementary school teacher

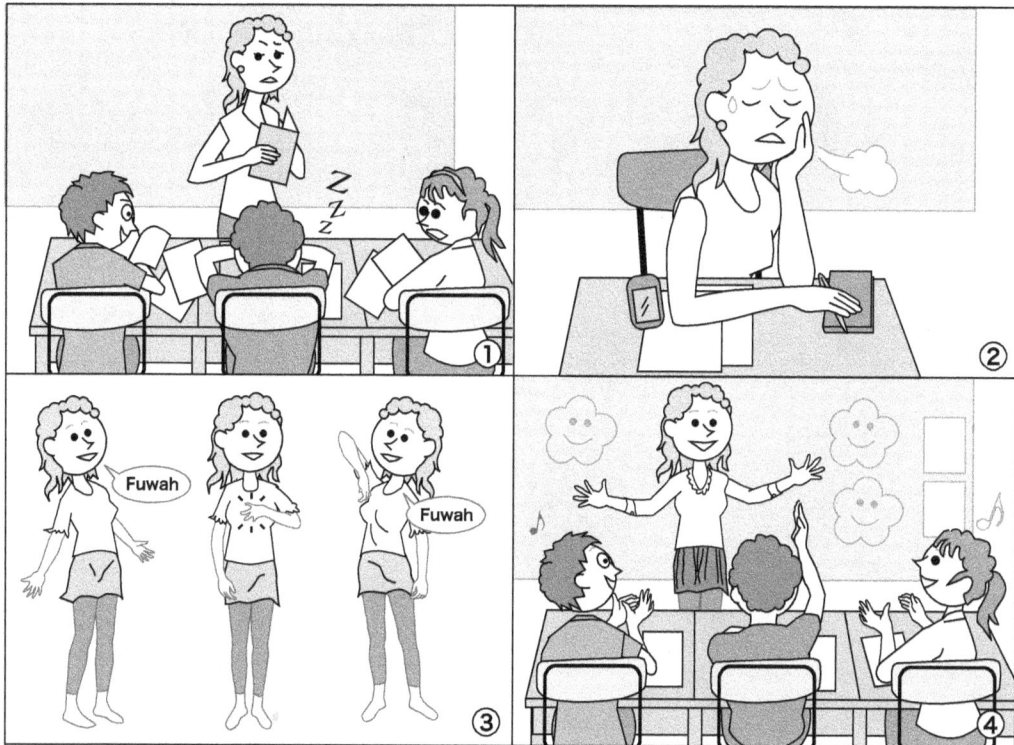

Sandra is an elementary school teacher. In her class, one student was sleeping. Another was reading a comic book. The others seemed bored with the class. She had become a teacher three years ago. Now the everyday work routine, the many complaints from parents,.... She was completely exhausted. She used to love teaching and had been full of energy and motivation. But not any more. It was all gone.

One day, she found a book talking about the YURU EXERCISES. She tried some of them. It made her body relaxed and her mind feel better. After she did the basic exercises, she tried the ones to develop the center and the lower tanden. She found that it gradually made her calmer. She could eliminate her problems and worries at work and take them easy. Next, she tried the exercise to develop the middle tanden, the source of passion. These helped her feel motivated. She liked the YURU EXERCISES and continued every single day.

A few weeks later, Sandra practiced the exercises before starting her class. She could feel something exciting. "Yes, this feeling is more like the one I used to have when I started teaching." The students felt her excitement and passion. They seemed to be joining the class with more fun and joy.

Arch
Ken: Researcher

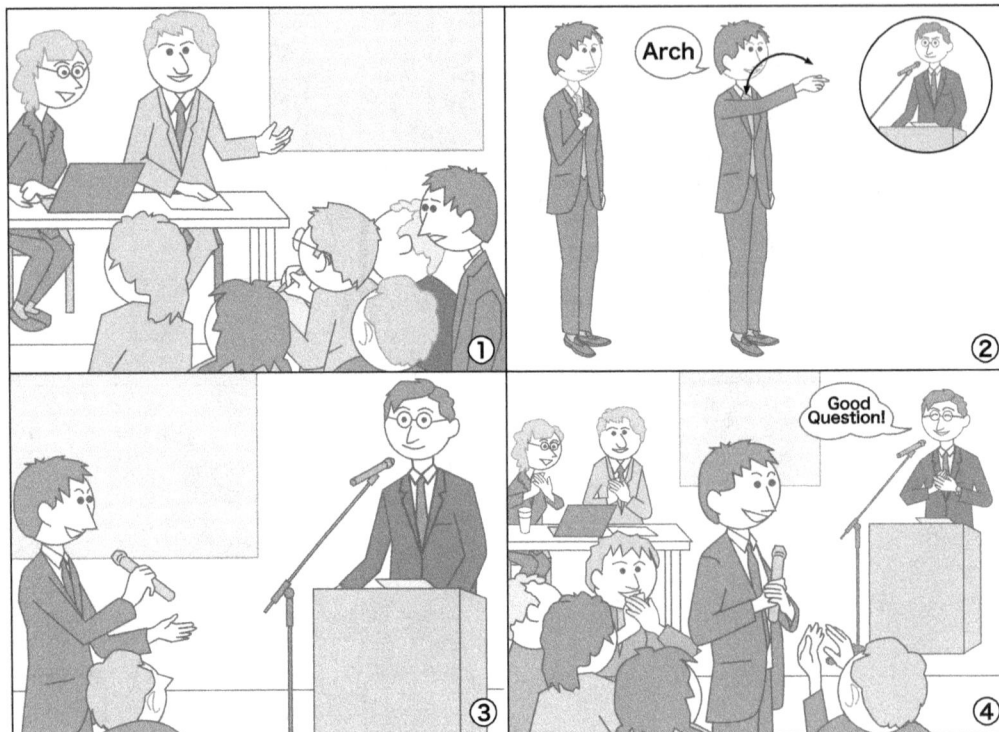

Ken is a young Japanese researcher. He attended an International conference which was held in English. He enjoyed participating in the conference and listening to the many interesting talks. He did not have any problems understanding English. However, speaking in public was totally different for him. He hated talking in front of many people. Especially when it's English, a language that is not his mother tongue.

At the end of the conference, there was a Q and A session. He had a question that he wanted to ask, but felt too shy to speak. So he walked to the back of the conference room where no one else was and repeated the arch towards the chairman. He gradually felt like he was connected to the chairman's heart.

He felt courage and went back to the main area. He raised his hand and spoke calmly. His question and points impressed everyone and the other participants praised him. He finally felt totally relaxed and had much more confidence about himself.

Vest (1)
Mary: Housewife

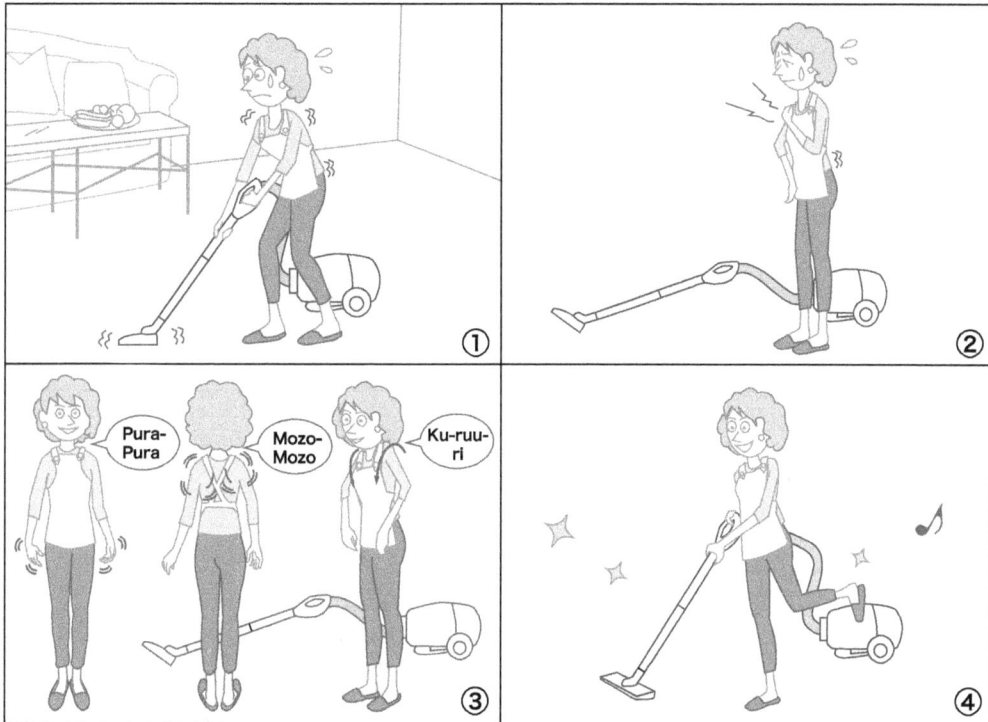

Mary is a housewife who doesn't like cleaning much. She was feeling lazy especially about vacuuming. It made her arms ache. She always tended to hold a vacuum cleaner too tight and push it on the floor too hard because she thought that's the way.

One day, a thought came to her mind. "Maybe the YURU EXERCISES to develop the vest work for this!"

First, she shook her wrists well and moved her shoulder blades to loosen them up. Next, she rolled her shoulders slowly and completely. She imagined that her arms and torso were more relaxed and flexible. She moved her arms from the far inside of her shoulder blades while vacuuming. She used to use her dominant hand mainly but she also tried using both arms equally. Rolling her shoulders. Switching her arms. While she was vacuuming she felt it's just like an exercise. It's fun. She discovered that no extra power was needed. She noticed that vacuuming required only minimum energy with a better body movement.

Vest (2)
David: Professional golfer

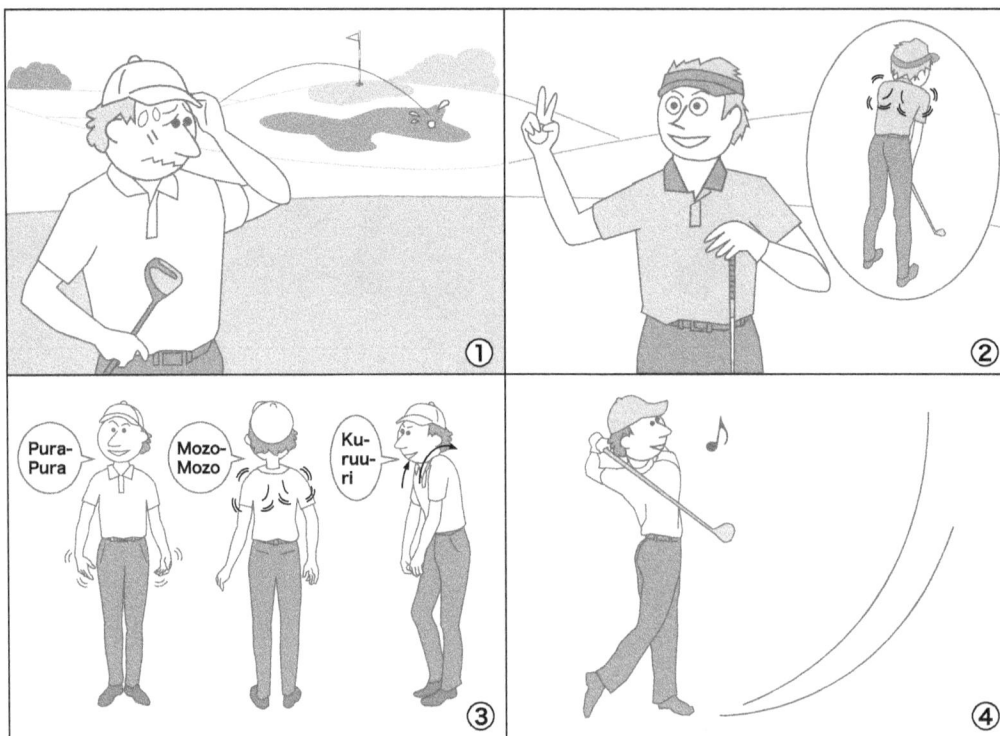

David is a professional golfer. He had won a championship but that was a long time ago when he was young. He is now in his 40s. Of course, he has more experience in golf now. His knowledge, technique, strategy,… everything has improved. But somehow his score has not been so good.

On the other hand, Tom, who became a professional golfer in the same year as David, seems to be in great condition. David asked Tom why he is in such good shape. Tom said he has been practicing YURU EXERCISES to develop his body awareness. "YURU EXERCISES?" "Yeah, it's in this new book I have on how to improve your body and mind at the same time--did you want to borrow it?" "Sure...."

"This is very interesting!" David incorporated the methods into his regular training menu. What he liked the most were the YURU EXERCISES to develop his vest. He found that it worked very well with the combination of the WRIST Pura-Pura EXERCISE and the SHOULDER BLADE Mozo-Mozo EXERCISE. It allowed him to use his arms broadly, made his swing more powerful, and extended his tee off distance dramatically. He also felt that he could shoot more accurately. Even better was he noticed that his shoulders were not stiff anymore but completely loosened up. He could also feel very relaxed mentally.

David will play in an upcoming championship soon. He now knows how to relax his body and mind. He can use his muscles well from deep inside his body. If he stays calm and just focuses on each shot, the results will follow.

Uratenshi
Linda: Project coordinator

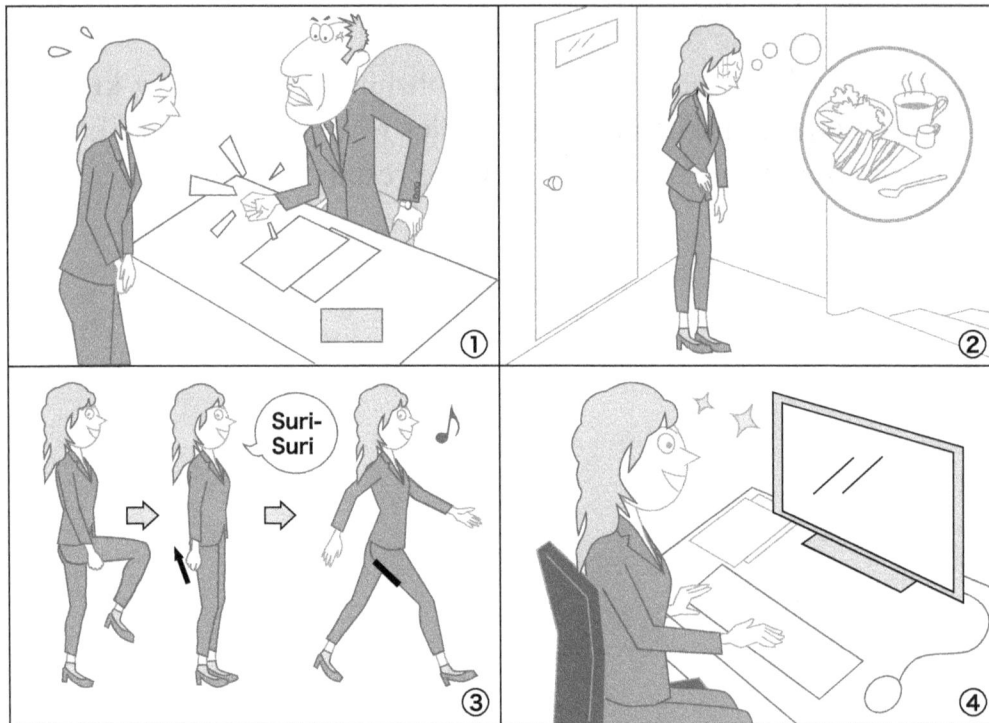

Linda is a project coordinator who works under huge pressure in a stressful environment. She was working very hard everyday but made one big mistake due to her carelessness. She wanted to convince herself that it was because of too much work. However, she knew that an excuse does not resolve anything.

She felt depressed and tried to go out of the office for lunch and to get some fresh air. Her eyes were looking down at the ground. Her back was curved forward. Her chest was tightly closed. Her legs were as heavy as rocks.

"No! I should not be like this. The past is past. I should look forward and act for now and the future." She rubbed her uratenshi and focused on it.

Her posture got better. She started walking more vigorously and gracefully. She felt refreshed and energized. Just walking, only changing her walking style made her feel better. After she got back to work from the lunch break, she felt more motivated and continued her work with a revitalized mind.

**Laser
Paul: CEO**

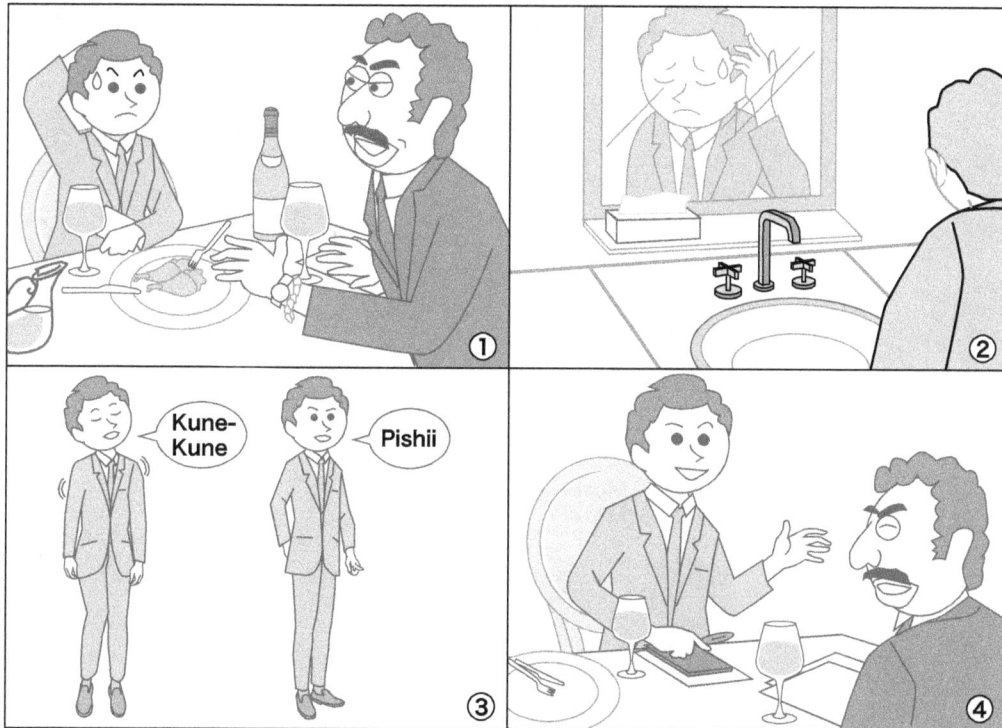

At a restaurant, Paul was undertaking a significant negotiation with his supplier, Bob. Bob is always very pushy. Paul was nervous and overwhelmed by him. The negotiation proceeded completely at Bob's pace.

Paul stood up, excused himself from the table, and went to the rest room. "No, this is not going to work. I cannot accept his deal. It would be a losing situation for our business." He was struggling and worried.

But then, he remembered the YURU EXERCISES. He tried to loosen up his body. He found himself feeling better and more relaxed. He focused on his center, the middle tanden, and the arch while strengthening them. He also focused on the laser. It was very necessary for him to tell Bob what his requirements were clearly.

On the way back to the table, he kept reminding himself making the laser towards Bob. Paul sat at the table and continued the negotiation. He was much less nervous and talked to Bob calmly and imposingly. He first showed his understanding of Bob's demand, but he also told Bob what he needed as well. Paul's unshakable attitude quite impressed Bob. The flow of the negotiation changed. They started seeking for a win-win situation for both of their companies.

YURU EXERCISE - variation
(Shaking & Loosening)
Liz: Yoga practitioner

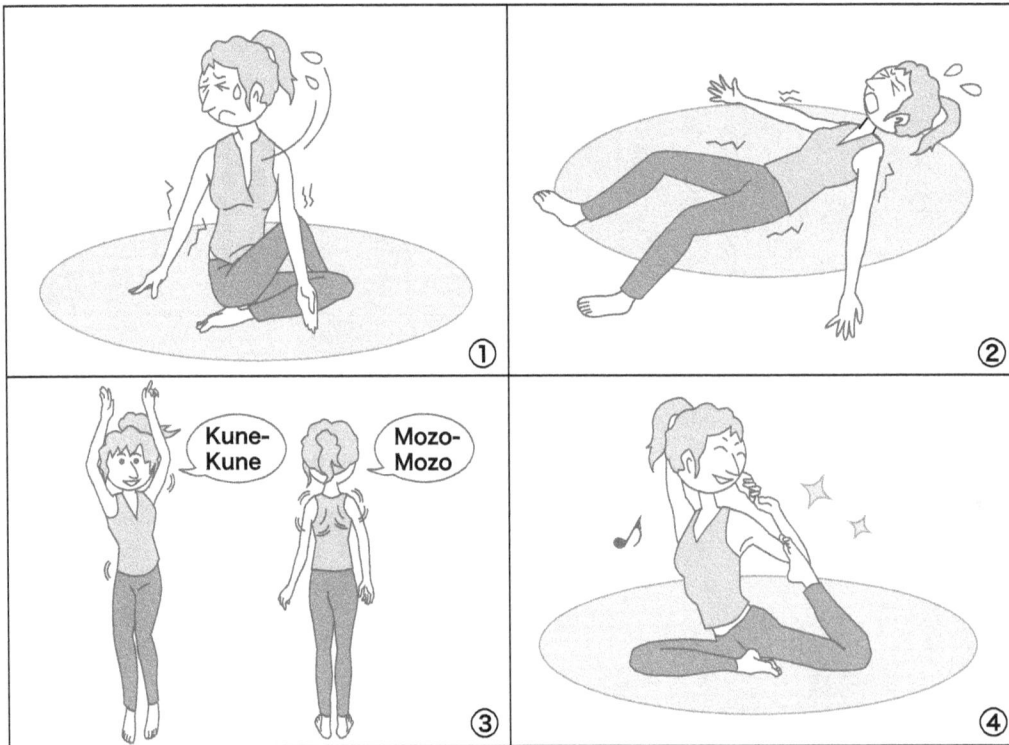

Liz has been practicing Yoga for five years. She has improved and become more flexible, but there was still room for improvement. Sometimes she pushed herself too hard and hurt her back and shoulders. She understood Yoga was not about pushing herself; not even about competing with others but she still wanted to have a breakthrough.

One day, she read a book about the YURU EXERCISES. "Shaking," "loosening," "humor," "onomatopoeia." These were things she hadn't been thinking about.

She tried to incorporate the YURU EXERCISES movements between poses during her Yoga practice. Deep and slow breathing is very important for Yoga. She did YURU movements softly and slowly while maintaining her breathing rhythm. She tried to carefully listen to her body to make sure she felt comfortable. It was a success. She found that the YURU shaking and loosening movements could make the transition of her postures smoother and easier. She successfully noticed that she could control her breathing, body, and mind more deeply and easily.

Conclusion

This book was written to reveal the secrets of the advanced abilities of the human body and to introduce you to various ways that can bring out such abilities hidden deep inside you. After you have read the book to the end, you might have noticed that this book also discusses the fundamental abilities of human beings for almost everyone that are beyond the mere physical capabilities of the body itself. That is the body awareness mechanism that exists deep inside your body and mind which is explained in this book.

I have introduced seven body awareness types including the center and the lower tanden. Body awareness is a factor that configures the structure of "the undifferentiated area of body and mind." From the late 19th to 20th centuries, the existence of such an area was assumed in the world of philosophy by centering on the theory of body.

However these philosophical studies could not reveal the structural functions of the body awareness. Certain structures exist in the undifferentiated area of the body and mind. There are many factors that generate that structure. High performances in our bodies and minds are supported by those factors and the structures. There were previously no findings with regard to these topics.

In my studies, I have mainly aimed to discover the structures and factors that exist in the undifferentiated area of the body and mind. I have also explored what kind of functions can be brought out through these structures and factors.

The above points have been gradually discovered in a wide range of areas in recent research. The kinds of abilities we can improve upon have also been revealed. In other words, we have discovered purposes we can aim at by training our body awareness. YURU EXERCISES is the ultimate effective training system. We have conducted a vast amount of educational experiments and studies. The YURU EXERCISES training system have been established and refined systematically by the training practiced by various people including athletes, musicians, performing artists, academic researchers, business people, doctors, teachers, students, housewives, etc.

In this book, I present the most representative structures and factors, the seven body awareness types and the training methods to develop those awarenesses, to the world for the first time. Even if you are not a professional athlete, if you engage in intellectual tasks for your work, study, or other endeavors, you can still use the

YURU EXERCISES. They can develop your body awareness and improve your work abilities and performance. They can greatly help your self improvement.

Furthermore you can use the YURU EXERCISES in unlimited areas related to your emotional, spiritual, and mental development as well as improvement of human relationships. For example, the center allows you to create a stable mental axis. The lower tanden lets you have a strong unshakable toughness even in critical situations. The middle tanden makes you more motivated and passionate. The arch strengthens and softens your relationships with others.

Therefore, the methods described in this book cannot only be used at home but also by people in various professional endeavors including medicine, care, education, production, distribution, information, and so on. Regardless of which field you belong to, for every area, for all fields, in all circumstances of your life, you can use the body awareness to fully improve your abilities and solve the problems that you face.

My greatest hope is that you will find value in the seven body awareness types from such a wide perspective and that you will gain full benefits from its theory and training routine, the YURU EXERCISES, to improve your life.

As mentioned in the Introduction chapter, we are currently working on the official website of YURU EXERCISES (http://yuruexercise.net/). It will provide you with many useful topics and information including features and benefits of YURU EXERCISES and medical scientific measurement data from the studies we have conducted. By presenting practical training videos and guidelines of teaching and studying instructions of YURU EXERCISES, this site will also be helpful for those who wish to practice YURU EXERCISES in full scale and those who wish to teach YURU EXERCISES.

You can get more information from another useful site, HIDEO TAKAOKA's GLOSSARIES that will be coming together with the YURU EXERCISES official site. Please visit these sites to enjoy more interesting and deeper knowledge of the YURU world and fully use it for your better health and life. (These sites are planned to open after October 2014.)

Lastly and most importantly, please keep in mind the following four key points on your body awareness training:

1) Before you try to develop your body awareness, loosen up every part of your body with the basic YURU EXERCISES that are common to all of body awareness types.
2) Loosen your body intensively, completely, and go further and deeper rather than just being relaxed.
3) To develop each of the seven body awareness types, be sure to create the center first and then work on the lower tanden.
4) When you practice the middle tanden, do not practice it excessively. Limit your practice to the maximum stated in this book.

I will end this book by sincerely wishing for your success and saying the above four points are the most important keys to develop your body awareness.

Hideo Takaoka

Acknowledgements

It is my great pleasure that the research and study I have conducted through the 40 years of my adult life have come to fruition and that I can deliver my knowledge and findings to you by publishing this book. This is because of all the guidance, support, understanding, and opportunities provided by many individuals and organizations around me who have been very supportive and cooperative. I would like to express my sincere gratitude especially to those whom I regard deeply in my heart.

My father, Tadashi Takaoka, was a proficient journalist at a major newspaper company as well as a private researcher who studied body and mind trainings all over the world. He taught me Japanese traditional martial arts that originated in the 14th century. It is considered historically as the highest level of martial arts in Japan. He also taught me Shinto, Buddhist Tantrism, Yoga, Taoism, Chinese martial arts, and the capabilities of animals. Both the education and problem consciousness that I obtained from him have always been the fundamental knowledge and motivations of my study, lifelong guidelines, as well as the research topics that I needed to pursue. In that sense, my father has been and always will be the greatest mentor of my entire life.

My mother, Ichi Takaoka, taught me about indestructible mental toughness, love, and devotion. She was an expert in living. Her house work was amazingly high level. In her life, she showed me, through her work, the many proofs that the concept of advanced mental and physical abilities could be acquired and exist not only for academics, arts or sports that people can easily recognize, but also for 'living' that is usually hidden from our thoughts.

My wife, Keiko Takaoka, is my important partner in both business and our private life. She is also the top student of the thousands of people I have instructed. One day, she came to my class. She was an ordinary piano teacher in town but had a strong hope to be able to play at the world's highest level even if just only for one piece. Since then, she has been beside me and has always supported me with her deep sincerity and love. She is my best example to prove the benefits of my training methods of body awareness development and breathing exercises including the YURU EXERCISES.

In my early childhood, I learned scientific insights and intellection from my eldest brother, Masaki Takaoka. His viewpoints and thinking were attractive to me and I fully enjoyed them. After I grew up, when I was in my late 20s, I was a graduate student of the University of Tokyo. It was the earliest days of my research and study. My second brother, Kazuo Takaoka, kindly supported me financially in order for me to continue my study. My elder sister, Hiroko Sugimoto, is a very sweet person being warm, simple, and saintly. I learned so many things from her wonderful personality. It is a salvation for me that she is always generous and accepted my free-wheeling lifestyle.

I am truly thankful to The University of Tokyo where I could conduct my studies for 15 years. There, I studied natural sciences such as biomechanics and kinesiology. What I learned in those days helped me to fundamentally develop and establish my basic theories of body awareness and YURU. I really appreciate the chief professor, Mitsumasa Miyashita, who provided me with guidance at that time. Great amounts of documentation research at the general library and at each department library; many discussions with researchers in each area of expertise; they were all helpful and valuable experiences for me to deepen my study.

It has been 30 years since I founded the Research Institute of Kinesiology that I now direct. During the first half of this period, I used all of my energy to bring up young researchers. I have never been able to forget about those days when thinking of today's achievements and success. Especially, Kiyoshi Sasaoka who is a religious scholar today and Takashi Saito who is a professor of Meiji University; these people were key players for accelerating the cultivation of the will and sense of ethics to educate people, the clarification of body awareness, and the development of various body trainings.

In my more recent time at the Institute, I have been very fortunate to be surrounded by excellent staff members who are truly sincere and very motivated. The significant advances in research, the striking development of various training methods, the active expansion of educational business, and the continuous writing and publication; these would not been possible without their efforts and help. In particular, Toru Sazawa, the executive director and chief of the secretariat of the Japan Yuru Association; Hitoshi Shimose, expert trainer of the educational business division; and Takamasa Yatabe, in charge of publication and design; their performance and success have been incredibly remarkable, especially Takamasa Yatabe's brilliant contributions were a great help for translating this book and our international publishing efforts.

I have written more than 100 books in Japan so far. When thinking about my life as an author, I feel deep gratitude to the publishing company who accepted and published my first book regarding martial arts and sports. It was 30 years ago. At that time, I was just a young graduate student. Keigado Publishing Co. Ltd. was a company who gave me the big chance to be an author. I would like to take this opportunity to express my deep appreciation to its president, Heizo Asada, and Kyoichi Asada for their kindness and support.

At last, I wish to express my gratitude to Babel Group for translating and publishing this book. I am hugely grateful to Miyoko Yuasa and Tomoki Hotta who provided me with the great opportunity to introduce the YURU EXERCISES to the world. The translator, Rieko Sasaki, conveyed this book's unique theory very adequately. She also provided me with many useful information and comments. Professor Peter Skaer gave us insightful advice from his expert viewpoint.

This has been a truly collaborative project which would never have happened without the invaluable, ongoing support of a talented and dedicated team. I would like to thank deeply all other people as well who worked on the production of this book.

Thank you all very much.

About the Author

Hideo Takaoka is a kinesiologist, the director of the Research Institute of Kinesiology, the developer of YURU, and the president and promotion committee member of the non-profit organization, Japan YURU Association.

YURU is Takaoka's complete dynamic training system to 'loosen up' the human body and mind. It consists of his unique theory, YURU THEORY, and practice methods, YURU PRACTICE. The YURU EXERCISES explained in this book are some of his training methods under the YURU PRACTICE. These exercises provide you with a strong mind, healthy living, and a highly effective body. Takaoka's well-balanced method is designed to train, improve, and grow the true nature of humans in all aspects of intelligence, emotions, and physical and mental ability throughout your entire life. He calls engaging in this training the YURU WAY.

Takaoka is also recognized throughout the sports, fitness, and health worlds in Japan as a professional writer who has written more than 100 books in the areas of martial arts, kinesiology, sports science, physical education, body awareness, advanced body mechanics, and natural life philosophy.

In his early childhood, his father, who continued the Japanese traditional martial arts that originated in Muromachi period in the 14th century, taught him martial arts. He grew up surrounded by the samurai culture.

In addition to the training and study of martial arts, he also dedicated his life to integration research and the study of eastern philosophy and western science regarding the human body and advanced abilities at the Graduate School of Education of the University of Tokyo where he received his master's degree. He has studied kinesiology profoundly. But unlike traditional kinesiology, Takaoka's study includes not just human or animal movements but also the body awareness of humans as well as the awareness hidden in a wide range of things including cultural products and assets, plants, minerals, and even the universe. Through his extensive study and research, he has revealed the true depth of body awareness—the fundamental essence which support human physical and mental abilities.

In Japanese martial arts, there have always been concepts of "sei-chu-sen (the center axis)", "hara (guts, intestinal fortitude)", etc. Takaoka found the key to discovering the existence of the body awareness from those concepts. "Sei-chu-sen" and "hara" are now introduced as "Center" and "Lower Tanden" respectively in this book.

After extensive studies including investigation of the above concepts, he revealed that the body awareness exists not only in the field of Japanese martial arts, but also in various other fields such as sports, physical cultures, performing arts, music, business, medicine, academia, and in many other areas. He has successfully discovered the full picture of its structures and functions.

He also studied a variety of physical training methods from all ages and cultures as well as the physical abilities of animals including, centrally, those of fish. The YURU EXERCISES were developed based on the theory and techniques of Japanese traditional martial arts. Together with the essence from those, multiple techniques are integrated including those to loosen and relax your body with body shaking and those to change your body dramatically using gentle humor and Japanese onomatopoeia.

The YURU EXERCISES are systematic methods that allow everybody to develop body awareness easily and effectively. Regardless of age or gender, many people have enjoyed and found groundbreaking benefits for their health, beauty, and advanced abilities from both the physical and mental aspects.

Takaoka currently provides guidance to top-level athletes, performing artists, musicians, actors, business owners, politicians and professors as well. The YURU EXERCISES have been very popular and widely practiced by many people from active top athletes to senior citizens.

After the 2011 Tohoku Earthquake, Takaoka was determined to support people in the disaster areas and direct the YURU EXERCISES project. He was involved in the teaching of the YURU EXERCISES for the victims' health maintenance and disease prevention.

Translator's Message

In the spring of last year, I was in Tokyo during the beautiful cherry blossom season. For a long time the author, Mr. Hideo Takaoka, had been training one of the most famous Japanese Kabuki actors in body awareness. Takaoka invited me to his student's Kabuki show so that I could gain better understanding of his theory through watching the student's performance. At that time, a year and a half had passed since I started working on Takaoka's translation project. I was thrilled to see the performance and excited to get further insight into the world of body awareness.

As you may know, Kabuki performers are required to wear heavy wigs and many layers of thick special kimonos. Can you imagine? Some of their costumes weigh more than 100 pounds! Even a lighter one is not very comfortable compared to the jeans and t-shirts we wear in daily life, or even any kind of sports uniform. Kabuki was originally started by a woman, but as time passed and due to historical reasons, all roles are now played by male performers. The actors playing female roles need to appear more feminine than females which require many types of body awareness, especially the highly developed center based on a completely loosened body.

The actor I saw was playing a young female. He was wearing a heavy wig and a very thick kimono with a tight belt. Furthermore, his body was constricted with many inner bands to prevent from the costume from becoming loose and untidy. I was told that the actor weighs about 150 pounds and his costume was about 110 pounds, which was around 75% of his body weight. Being physically strong is not enough to perform Kabuki well. Relying on just physical strength would make his movements awkward and he would waste his muscular power. It would be far different from movements that are described as elegant or feminine.

Despite such a heavy and constricting costume, the actor's performance was just incredible. His movements seemed very natural and elegant. His body usage had no awkward parts at all. Rather it was dynamic and fluid while at the same time soft and gentle. What I saw were just smooth, graceful, beautiful movements.

While watching the performance, I did not fully understand how the body awareness was used. But after the show, Takaoka explained how the actor's body awareness worked and what the actor had been learning, including the movement of his neck, back, spine, arms, legs, ... and even eye level. It was an absolutely wonderful experience to help me translate this book and also for my own body usage and for life itself.

Throughout this translation project, I was constantly trying to be aware of and develop my center and lower tanden. It helped me clear my mind and solve many issues that I faced with the language and culture differences. The laser was also an important key for me to focus on this job and complete it.

Translating Takaoka's words is always fun, especially after I met him in person and saw his great posture; just like a model. I really wanted to learn more about the body awareness. Actually, I learned much working on this project. I appreciate this opportunity to work with him and recommend mastering the body awareness to anybody who wishes to solve their problems and improve their strength physically, mentally, and emotionally.

Aside from Mr. Takaoka, there were other wonderful experts who kindly and greatly helped me in this project. Mr. Takamasa Yatabe, Takaoka's assistant, who knows Takaoka's theory very well, taught me many key points of Takaoka's exercise methods. He was always providing me with all sorts of additional information in a very professional manner, sometimes with a lot of humor, and at other times with his sincerity. It was so much fun working with him. He is one who has absolutely obtained all of the seven body awareness types.

The editor, Prof. Peter Skaer of Hiroshima University Japan, is truly my respected teacher. His insights and viewpoints were always very sharp and sophisticated. Compared to the original Japanese version of this book, this English book has a great deal of new content and revisions to accommodate readers worldwide. Without Prof. Skaer's help, it would not have been possible.

I cannot complete this message without mentioning the tremendous help of all members of the Babel group who were involved in this project. Their contributions were always appreciated. I would like to express my gratitude to them from the bottom of my heart.

At last, I wish to say thank you to all of you readers. I hope you find many benefits from this book and will become more and more interested in the body awareness.

Body awareness changes your habits! Your habits change your life!!
Let's be relaxed and loosened! Live better and healthier!!

Rieko Sasaki

www.ingramcontent.com/pod-product-compliance
Lightning Source LLC
Chambersburg PA
CBHW080849300326
41935CB00040B/1650